Contents

Preface

The prospect of facing examinations in psychiatry may be daunting and conjure up feelings of dread and panic, especially if one is under-prepared. As with other medical specialties, there are numerous facts that need to be digested within a short-time frame and this may seem like an endless process.

In recent years, there has been an increasing trend towards the use of extended matching questions (EMQs) and objective structured clinical examinations (OSCEs) as a method of assessment. This has been the case in many medical school final examinations, as well as postgraduate examinations such as the membership examination of the Royal College of Psychiatrists and the Professional and Linguistic Assessment Board (PLAB) examination. Unlike the traditional multiple choice question papers and clinical long cases, EMQs are thought to mirror clinical decision-making skills and OSCEs allow the standardisation of patients so that every candidate is marked objectively against the same criteria.

Although there are many good psychiatry textbooks available that cover the subject comprehensively, few books are dedicated to revision for examinations in the updated format. This book covers a broad range of topics in the form of EMQs and OSCEs, and will help the reader apply theoretical knowledge to common clinical situations. It will be essential in preparing for examinations, and will be a great supplement to larger textbooks.

Many of the questions in this book were developed through teaching and testing medical students, who were very patient and kind enough to make suggestions. This book is aimed primarily for medical students, as dedicated psychiatry revision textbooks at their level are in great demand. It will also be helpful for oversea doctors studying for the PLAB examinations, and may appeal to the trainee psychiatrist as a refresher.

As with any other examinations, practice is the key to doing well in psychiatry examinations, and the authors hope that this book will serve as a stepping stone in shaping your revision. We hope that you will enjoy learning about psychiatry and wish you lots of luck with your examinations.

Kazuya Iwata
Afia Ali

List of Abbreviations

AA	Alcoholics Anonymous
ACE	Angiotensin converting enzyme
ADH	Antidiuretic hormone
ADHD	Attention-deficit/hyperactivity disorder
AIDS	Acquired immunodeficiency syndrome
AOT	Assertive outreach team
APA	American Psychiatric Association
ASW	Approved social worker
BMI	Body mass index
CAT	Cognitive analytical therapy
CBT	Cognitive behavioural therapy
CDAT	Community drugs and alcohol team
CJD	Creutzfeldt–Jakob disease
CMHT	Community mental health team
CNS	Central nervous system
CPA	Care programme approach
CPMS	Clozaril Patient Monitoring Service
CRT	Crisis resolution team
CSF	Cerebrospinal fluid
CT	Computer tomography
CVA	Cerebrovascular accident
DBT	Dialectical behavioural therapy
DSH	Deliberate self-harm
DSM-IV	Diagnostic and Statistical Manual of Mental Disorders, Fourth Edition
DVLA	Driver and Vehicle Licensing Agency
ECG	Electrocardiogram
ECT	Electroconvulsive therapy
ED	Emergency Department
EEG	Electroencephalogram
EIS	Early intervention services
EMDR	Eye movement desensitisation and reprocessing
EPSE	Extra-pyramidal side effects
FSH	Follicular-stimulating hormone
GABA	Gamma aminobutyric acid

GHB	Gamma hydroxybutyric acid
GP	General practitioner
HIV	Human immunodeficiency virus
HPA	Hypothalamic–pituitary–adrenal axis
ICD-10	International Statistical Classification of Diseases and Related Health Problems, Tenth Revision
IQ	Intelligence quotient
LFT	Liver function test
LH	Luteinising hormone
LSD	Lysergic acid diethylamide
MAOI	Monoamine oxidase inhibitor
MDMA	3,4-Methylenedioxy-N-methylamphetamine
MHA	Mental Health Act of England and Wales, 1983
MMSE	Mini-mental state examination
MRI	Magnetic resonance imaging
NaRI	Noradrenaline reuptake inhibitor
NaSSA	Noradrenergic and specific serotonergic antidepressant
NICE	UK National Institute for Health and Clinical Excellence
NMDA	N-methyl-D-aspartic acid
NSAID	Non-steroidal anti-inflammatory drug
OCD	Obsessive-compulsive disorder
OT	Occupational therapist
PANSS	Positive and negative syndrome scale
PICU	Psychiatric Intensive Care Unit
REM	Rapid eye movement
RMO	Responsible medical officer
SFRS	Schneiderian first-rank symptom
SNRI	Serotonin–noradrenaline reuptake inhibitor
SSRI	Selective serotonin reuptake inhibitor
TSH	Thyroid-stimulating hormone
WHO	World Health Organisation

Introduction

This book contains 58 EMQs divided into eight chapters according to topics for ease of revision. Each EMQ has 10 items and five statements. Each statement has only one possible answer and each item is used only once. There are several styles to the questions, but they are usually based on a clinical vignette to assist application of knowledge to clinical situations. Some factual questions are also included. Each question is followed by a detailed explanation of the answers and useful teaching notes. The questions vary in the degree of difficulty, but the overall difficulty is titrated to moderate level. Some challenging questions are also included to test the more knowledgeable students aiming for distinction. Deliberate repetitions of similar concepts are made to emphasise their importance. The last EMQ chapter contains questions that have been grouped by clinical presentation and is therefore more likely to reflect the actual examination and clinical situation.

The OSCE section comprises of 23 common clinical situations that are likely to be encountered in clinical examination situations. The introductory section gives general advice on approaching OSCE stations, and this is followed by sample OSCE marking schemes. It is suggested that these marking schemes be used as a framework in structuring the approach to each station.

The book primarily refers to the *Tenth Revision of the International Statistical Classification of Diseases and Related Health Problems (ICD-10)* published by the World Health Organisation (WHO) in defining mental illnesses, but clinical descriptions from the *Diagnostic and Statistical Manual of Mental Disorders, Fourth Edition (DSM-IV)* published by the American Psychiatric Association (APA) are also included. Although diagnostic concepts are discussed in this book, those who are interested in learning the actual diagnostic criteria for individual mental illnesses should refer to the appropriate chapters in the ICD-10 (WHO) and DSM-IV (APA).

Where legislations and guidelines are involved, references are made to those that are in wide use in England and Wales. To this end, references are made to the 1983 Mental Health Act of England and Wales (MHA) in discussing mental health legislations and compulsory admissions to hospital. In discussing the management of mental illnesses, clinical guidelines issued by the UK National Institute for Health and Clinical Excellence (NICE) are followed. With regards to substance use, alcohol measurements are made in units, which is widely used in the UK for alcohol consumption approximation. References are made to the UK Misuse of Drug Act in classifying illegal substances. Readers are encouraged to keep themselves updated with any changes in such legislations and guidelines.

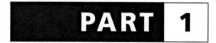

PART 1

Extended matching questions (EMQs)

The following EMQs contain 10 choices (A–J) followed by five numbered statements. For each stem, select the single best choice that best corresponds to the given information. Each stem has only *one* answer, and each choice can be used only *once*.

CHAPTER 1

Introduction to psychiatry

Acronyms in psychiatry

A. ASW
B. CPA
C. DSM
D. EPSE
E. ICD
F. MHA
G. MMSE
H. PANSS
I. PICU
J. RMO

Select the most appropriate item from the above that is best defined by the following statements.

1. The fourth edition of this classification system of mental disorders devised by the American Psychiatric Association assesses patients on five dimensions.

2. A useful bedside tool used in assessing the patient's cognition on a 30-point scale.

3. Framework of aftercare of discharged patients in England and Wales, identified through a coordinated multidisciplinary assessment of patient's health and social care needs.

4. Defines mental disorder as 'mental illness, arrested or incomplete development of mind, psychopathic disorder, and any other disorder or disability of mind.'

5. A group of side effects of antipsychotic medications, including parkinsonism, tardive dyskinesia, akathisia, and acute dystonia.

Important names in psychiatry

A. Described schizophrenia as being associated with auditory hallucinations and made affect.

B. Described the classic symptoms of schizophrenia to include delusional perception and thought echo.

C. Described the classic symptoms of schizophrenia to include loosening of association and ambivalence.

D. Described schizophrenia as being associated with thought broadcast and incongruous affect.

E. Described schizophrenia as being type I (acute) and type II (chronic).

F. Explained that the underlying dysfunctional beliefs of depression include negative views of the self, the world, and the future.

G. Focused on the cognitive model of schizoaffective disorder.

H. Identified that 'early maternal loss' and 'lack of confiding relationship' as vulnerability factors for the development of depression.

I. Identified that high expressed emotions play a role in the aetiology of schizophrenia.

J. Through animal experiments, found that love and comfort is necessary for attachment.

Select the most appropriate item from the above that is best associated with the following names.

1. Brown and Harris

2. Kurt Schneider

3. Eugene Bleuler

4. Aaron Beck

5. TJ Crow

Mental state examination I

A. Appearance
B. Behaviour
C. Thought form and speech
D. Mood
E. Affect
F. Thought content
G. Abnormal perception
H. Cognition
I. Insight
J. Not part of mental state examination

The following were obtained during a clinical interview with a patient. Select the most appropriate choice from the above where you would record the information obtained.

1. 'I don't know what to do, doctor. I know that they are monitoring my actions using special radio waves and there's no way I can get away from it.'

2. 'Can't you hear them? They're constantly criticising me.'

3. 'I'm not eating anymore, and I constantly feel guilty for everything. I feel like I'm in a deep trench and I'm suffering down below.'

4. 'After that, I decided to go home ... Home and away ... Swaying my way.'

5. 'I don't need these tablets ... Everything that is happening to me is real! I'm not mad and I'm definitely not staying in hospital.'

Mental state examination II

A. Alexithymia
B. Anhedonia
C. Blunting of affect
D. Circumstantiality
E. Delusional mood
F. Incongruity of mood
G. Knight's move thinking
H. Labile mood
I. Perseveration
J. Tangentiality

The following were obtained during a clinical interview with a patient. Select the most appropriate item from the above that best describes the clinical presentations depicted.

1. 'My uncle got killed in a car accident 2 days ago. Ha ha. He was speeding and the car just went out of control!!! Ha ha ha ... I can't stop laughing!'

2. 'I don't really do the things that I used to do. I used to be an active person and enjoyed running. I even played tennis competitively and really liked it, but they don't seem to be pleasurable at all. I don't get any joy out of my hobbies now.'

3. 'You want to know where I'm from? That's a hard question because I'm technically from the UK but I do know that my ancestors came from northern Europe. I think several generations ago they were living as Vikings. But yes, I'm from England.'

4. 'It just feels so strange. I know something weird is going on and that something will definitely happen soon. I can't exactly explain it, but I know it's going to be horrible.'

5. 'Yes I do take my medications as directed, doctor. I take one tablet every morning after having my breakfast, and then it was his turn to be punished. It's a fight involving everyone, but the unaffected third party just pretended nothing happened.'

Psychiatric phenomenology I

A. Autochthonous delusion
B. Delusional atmosphere
C. Delusional memory
D. Delusional perception
E. Depersonalisation
F. Derealisation
G. Echo de la pensee
H. Secondary delusion
I. Somatic passivity
J. Thought insertion

Select the most appropriate item from the above that best matches the clinical description in the following statements.

1. A patient goes out shopping. While waiting at the checkout counter, he suddenly feels empty and detached from the rest of the world, as if his soul was outside his body and overlooking everything.

2. A patient goes out shopping. While waiting at the checkout counter, it dawns on to him that he was the Son of God. He subsequently stands on top of the counter and starts screaming religious chants to convince others of his divine status.

3. A patient goes out shopping. While waiting at the checkout counter, he finds an old coin in his wallet, which he thought he had previously lost. He then knew that he was the Son of God.

4. A patient goes out shopping. While waiting at the checkout counter, he thought he heard someone say, 'You're the Son of God!' but could not find anyone around him. He concludes that a divine being must be talking to him, and is now convinced he is God.

5. A patient goes out shopping. While waiting at the checkout counter, he claims that there are special radio waves transmitted in the air that are planting ideas in his mind that he was the Son of God.

Psychiatric phenomenology II

A. Elementary hallucination
B. Extracampine hallucination
C. Functional hallucination
D. Hypnagogic hallucination
E. Hypnopompic hallucination
F. Illusion
G. Pseudohallucination
H. Second-person auditory hallucination
I. Third-person auditory hallucination
J. Thought echo

Select the most appropriate item from the above that best matches the clinical description in the following statements.

1. A 15-year-old female is walking along the street at night and mistakes the shadow of a tree as a man holding a gun.

2. A 20-year-old male with schizophrenia feels distressed as he constantly hears several voices talking to each other about his actions and thoughts right behind him, saying: 'Look at him, he's a loser.'

3. A 25-year-old female can hear the voice of her dead mother in her head reading a poem. She knows the voices are not real, but feels distressed by it.

4. A 34-year-old male claims that he can hear buzzing noises in the background and see lights flashing before his eyes.

5. A 16-year-old female is worried that she can hear her name being called out when she is falling asleep.

Psychiatric phenomenology III

A. Delusion of control
B. Delusion of jealousy
C. Delusion of guilt
D. Delusion of reference
E. Delusion of thought interference
F. Erotomanic (amorous) delusion
G. Grandiose delusion
H. Hypochondriacal delusion
I. Nihilistic delusion
J. Persecutory delusion

The following scenarios refer to a patient with delusional ideas. Select the single most appropriate item from the above that best matches the type of delusion depicted.

1. A 23-year-old male believes that his life and the world are coming to an end after having lost his job. He has stopped looking after himself and has not eaten in 3 days as he believes that his body organs are decaying.

2. A 19-year-old male is terrified because he feels that his actions and feelings are no longer his own. He believes that a device is making him think in negative ways and do things that are embarrassing, as if he was a robot.

3. A 26-year-old female has been living on the streets for the last week because she knows that a famous actor is planning a vendetta to kill her. She feels unsafe wherever she goes as she feels that she is constantly under threats of an attack.

4. A 30-year-old female cleaner was brought to hospital for trying to set fire to her garden. She insists that the newspapers contain articles with covert messages criticising her garden and thus decided to set fire in order to build a new one.

5. A 28-year-old male doctor believes that he is the best looking male in the world and that everyone at work is trying to befriend him. He also claims that he is highly gifted and that he had cured his own leukaemia.

Answers

Acronyms in psychiatry

1. **C.** DSM stands for *Diagnostic and Statistical Manual for Mental Disorders*, published by the American Psychiatric Association. The most recent edition is the fourth edition (DSM-IV). It is a multi-axial diagnostic system using five axes, meaning that the diagnoses of a patient are coded into five categories or axes:
   - Axis I describes clinical psychiatric disorders.
   - Axis II describes any personality disorders or mental retardation.
   - Axis III describes general medical conditions.
   - Axis IV describes current psychosocial problems.
   - Axis V is a global assessment of functioning using a scale.

2. **G.** MMSE stands for the mini-mental state examination, which is a bedside tool used in assessing cognition with a 30-point scale, covering orientation, registration, concentration, recall, language, and praxis. A score of 27–30 is considered normal.

3. **B.** CPA stands for Care Programme Approach. This was introduced in 1991 in England and Wales to ensure that there is adequate provision of services and regular monitoring of people with mental illness who have been discharged into the community. The purpose is to provide support for individuals, to improve continuity of care, and to maximise the effects of any therapeutic intervention.

4. **F.** The 1983 Mental Health Act of England and Wales has a broad definition of mental disorder. It essentially includes those with a mental illness or a learning disability. Psychopathic disorder is a legal term, with dissocial personality disorder being the nearest psychiatric diagnosis. Specific 'sections' of the MHA allow detention of patients in mental health units for assessment and treatment purposes.

5. **D.** EPSE stands for extra-pyramidal side effects, which are movement-related side effects seen with the use of dopamine antagonists such as antipsychotics. These include acute dystonia, akathisia, parkinsonism, and tardive dyskinesia. All of them are reversible upon cessation of the antidopaminergic medications or through the use of anticholinergic medications (such as procyclidine), apart from tardive dyskinesia.

Notes

- RMO stands for Responsible Medical Officer, who is usually the consultant.

- ICD-10 is the International Statistical Classification of Diseases and Health Related Problems, 10th Edition, published by the World Health Organisation. This is the classification guide that lists all medical conditions, and the section on psychiatric illnesses is used as the basis of classification of psychiatric illnesses in the UK.

- PICU stands for Psychiatric Intensive Care Unit, where patients who cannot be managed in an open ward because of aggression or risk of absconding are managed.

- ASW stands for Approved Social Worker, who is specially trained to assess patients under the 1983 Mental Health Act of England and Wales.

- PANSS stands for Positive and Negative Syndrome Scale, which is a rating tool commonly used to rate symptoms of psychotic illnesses.

Important names in psychiatry

1. **H.** Brown and Harris's study in Camberwell, London (1978) showed that the following factors increased the vulnerability to depression in women:
   - Lack of a confiding relationship.
   - Unemployment.
   - Three or more children under the age of 14 years.
   - Loss of mother before the age of 11 years.

2. **B.** In order to differentiate schizophrenia from other psychotic illnesses, Kurt Schneider listed the first-rank symptoms of schizophrenia as being central features of schizophrenia, but not necessary for its diagnosis. There are 11 Schneiderian first-rank symptoms (SFRS), which can be broadly categorised into four groups as follows:
   - Delusional perception.
   - Thought insertion, thought withdrawal, thought broadcast.
   - Third-person auditory hallucinations, hallucinations in the form of a running commentary, thought echo.
   - Somatic passivity, and passivity of affect, impulse, and volition.

3. **C.** Bleuler listed the four A's to describe schizophrenia: ambivalence, affective abnormalities, loosening of association, and autism.

4. **F.** Beck's cognitive triad of depression refers to a negative view of the self, the world, and the future.

5. **E.** Crow described two types of schizophrenia:
   - Type I schizophrenia has an acute onset, comprises of positive symptoms, and responds well to antipsychotics with a good prognosis. He made the assumption that the brain was structurally normal.
   - Type II schizophrenia has a chronic onset, comprises of negative symptoms, and responds poorly to antipsychotics with a poor prognosis. There is an abnormal brain structure (cortical atrophy and ventricular dilatation).

Notes
- Harlow conducted an experiment on monkeys and found that baby monkeys formed attachment to comfortable but milkless dolls that offered comfort and security rather than metallic dolls that provided milk.

- Studies by Brown showed that high levels of expressed emotion can worsen the prognosis of those with mental illnesses.

Mental state examination I
1. **F.** Any notable content of thought should be recorded here, including the presence of delusions, obsessive thoughts, and phobias. A risk assessment should also be conducted to assess for any ideations of harming self or others. This is particularly important for those presenting with self-harm to ascertain the presence of any active suicidal ideation.

2. **G.** Any visual, auditory, olfactory, gustatory, tactile, and somatic illusions and hallucinations are recorded under 'abnormal perceptions'.

3. **D.** Features of subjective (patient's own words) and objective (as observed in interview) mood should be recorded under 'mood', including any associated biological features such as the effect of mood on appetite and sleep.

4. C. This is an example of flight of ideas, which is a rapid succession of thoughts vaguely associated with the sounds of other words. There may be punning and rhyming. This commonly occurs in patients with mania and is a disorder of the form of speech.

- Loosening of association occurs in schizophrenia, and this includes 'knight's move thinking' where there is no logical association between successive thoughts, 'word salad' where speech is an incomprehensible mixture of words and phrases, and 'neologisms' where a new word is invented by the patient.

5. I. Assessment of insight involves identifying whether the patient believes that he or she has an illness, whether the illness is attributed to a mental disorder, whether the patient believes that psychiatric treatment will be helpful, and whether they are willing to accept advice.

Mental state examination II

1. F. Incongruity of mood is the dissociation of one's emotions and the content of one's thoughts or actions. The observed affect is inappropriate to the situation, such as laughing when talking about something that is normally perceived as being sad.

2. B. Anhedonia is loss of enjoyment in previously pleasurable activities and interests. It is a core feature of depression.

3. D. Circumstantiality is a type of disorder of thought form (formal thought disorder) in which the patient goes at verbose length to include every detail in order to answer a simple question. In the course of the response, the eventual answer to the question is reached.

4. E. Delusional mood (also known as delusional atmosphere) is a type of primary delusion where the patient feels that something odd is going on or is about to happen.

5. G. Knight's move thinking is a type of formal thought disorder in which the patient starts answering the question appropriately, but the line of thought is suddenly shifted to an unrelated topic. It is also known as derailment of thought.

- Tangentiality is a related formal thought disorder in which the patient starts answering the question, but then talks off the topic in an area that is only indirectly related to the intended answer ('talking off the point'). As a result, the answer to the original question is not reached.

Notes

- Alexithymia refers to the inability to describe one's subjective emotional state. For example, an alexithymic individual would not be able to verbalise his sad and low feelings despite feeling so. It is also seen in somatisation disorder.

- Emotional blunting refers to a lack of emotional sensitivity and loss of appropriate responses to events that would usually invoke a response. It is a negative symptom of schizophrenia. Similarly, flattening of affect refers to a marked decrease in the usual range of emotions. It may be seen in a severely depressed patient who no longer feels the will to live and finds nothing interesting, or in a patient with schizophrenia.

- A labile mood indicates a marked variability in the affect, with rapid changes in mood observed over a short period of time, for example crying and then suddenly laughing within a minute.

- Perseveration is the inability to switch from one line of thinking to another. An example of this is when a patient who is asked about his family history continues to talk about this even when the doctor asks him about his social history.

Psychiatric phenomenology I

1. **E.** Depersonalisation is a subjective experience where the patient feels as if he or she is not real. It is a dream-like state experienced also by normal people.

2. **A.** A delusion is a fixed and unshakeable abnormal belief that is held with conviction and is out of keeping with the patient's cultural and religious background. An autochthonous delusion is a primary delusion and arises 'out of the blue'. A primary delusion occurs as a direct result of psychopathology.

3. **D.** Delusional perception is the perception of a normal object, in this case a coin, which is misinterpreted and given a delusional meaning (Son of God). This is also a type of primary delusion and is a first-rank symptom of schizophrenia.

4. **H.** Secondary delusions occur secondary to other psychopathology or psychiatric conditions. In this case the patient developed a delusion after hearing an auditory hallucination of a voice.

5. **J.** Thought insertion is a first-rank symptom of schizophrenia whereby the patient believes that thoughts are being placed inside the head by an outside source and that they are clearly not his or her own thoughts. Other thought-related delusions are thought broadcast, thought withdrawal, and thought echo (also known as echo de la pensee), which are all first-rank symptoms as well.

Notes
• Delusional atmosphere, also known as delusional mood, is a type of primary delusion in which the patient develops an uneasy feeling that something strange is going on around them or is about to happen.

• Derealisation is a phenomenon related to depersonalisation, but the unreal quality is associated with the world (as opposed to themselves). It has an 'as if' quality, for example 'as if everything around me was made from cardboard.'

• Somatic passivity is a subtype of delusion of control, in which the individual feels that specific body sensations are being controlled and enforced on them by an outside influence.

Psychiatric phenomenology II
1. **F.** An illusion is an abnormal perception in the *presence* of an external stimulus. On the other hand, a hallucination is an abnormal perception in the *absence* of an external stimulus.

2. **I.** Third-person auditory hallucinations are voices that refer to the patient as 'he' or 'she'. When commenting or discussing the patient, it is a first-rank symptom of schizophrenia.

3. G. Pseudohallucinations can be defined in two ways. The first definition is that of a false perception occurring *within* the person's mind, for example 'hearing voices in my head'. The second definition is that of a true hallucination, but the patient acknowledges them as being unreal and false, for example a widower hearing the voice of her dead husband but acknowledging it as being unreal.

4. A. An elementary hallucination is a type of hallucination that occurs in a very simple form such as hearing a buzzing sound or seeing flashes of light. It is more likely to occur in organic disease.

5. D. A hypnagogic hallucination is a transient experience that occurs on the verge of falling asleep, while hypnopompic hallucinations occur while waking up. They can both occur in normal people.

Notes

• An extracampine hallucination occurs when the origin of the percept occurs outside the range of normal senses, for example a patient claiming to hear a lecture being given in a class located 20 miles away.

• A functional hallucination is a hallucination that is only experienced when there is a normal perception in that same modality, for example hearing voices only when a water tap is heard running.

• A second-person auditory hallucination occurs when the patient hears voices talking directly to the patient and refers to the patient as 'you'. It is common in psychotic depression.

• Thought echo (also known as echo de la pensee) refers to a phenomenon where patients can hear their own thoughts spoken out loud as they think.

Psychiatric phenomenology III

1. I. A nihilistic delusion is marked with gloom and pessimism, in that the patient believes that they are dying or dead, or alternatively the world is coming to an end.

2. A. A delusion of control comprises several subtypes, but the core delusion is that one's body is no longer under one's control.

It is also known as passivity phenomena, and divided into passivity of affect (feelings), passivity of volition (actions), passivity of impulse, and somatic passivity (bodily sensations).

3. J. A persecutory delusion refers to a delusion whereby one believes that one's own life is being interfered or at danger because of another person or organisation. It is commonly thought to be synonymous to a paranoid delusion, but strictly speaking, a paranoid delusion applies to any delusion referring to one's self and thus includes any subtypes such as persecutory, grandiose, hypochondriacal, etc.

4. D. A delusion of reference is a delusion in which the individual believes that external events have special messages or relevance aimed specifically at him or her, for example television programmes making references to them.

5. G. A grandiose delusion is a delusion whereby the patient believes that he or she has special powers, wealth, or high social status. It is commonly seen in the manic phase of bipolar affective disorder.

Notes
- Delusion of jealousy (also known as morbid jealousy) involves the patient believing that one's spouse or partner is unfaithful despite very little evidence supporting this. It is commonly seen in the context of chronic alcohol abuse.

- Delusion of guilt is a delusion in which the patient holds a strong sense of guilt and shame as they believe they have committed a crime or misdemeanour in the past.

- Delusion of thought interference involves the patient believing that their own thoughts are under the influence of an external source, and refers to delusions of thought withdrawal, thought insertion, and thought broadcast.

- Erotomanic (amorous) delusion is a delusion in which the patient (usually female) believes that an individual, usually of a higher social status, is in love with them.

- Hypochondriacal delusion refers to a delusion in which the patient believes that he or she suffers from a specific medical illness, usually a severe, chronic illness such as cancer or HIV.

CHAPTER 2

General adult psychiatry

Psychotic illness I

A. Acute and transient psychotic disorder
B. Bipolar affective disorder
C. Catatonic schizophrenia
D. Hebephrenic schizophrenia
E. Paranoid schizophrenia
F. Residual schizophrenia
G. Schizoaffective disorder
H. Schizotypal disorder
I. Simple schizophrenia
J. Undifferentiated schizophrenia

The following patients present with a psychotic episode. Select the most appropriate diagnosis from the above that best fits with the following clinical description.

1. An 18-year-old male is brought to hospital by his parents because they have noticed that he has been acting strangely recently. His parents say that the patient has just 'lost it' since failing his final examinations. The patient was noted to be giggling to himself, spending almost all his time in his room, and making unusual gestures with his hands. In addition, his speech has been incomprehensible and his parents cannot make any sense of it.

2. A 30-year-old female is brought to hospital as she has been violent and hostile to her neighbours. According to the patient, her grandfather was a successful writer and she acquired his fortunes recently. However, she believes that her neighbours have found out about it and claims that she has heard them talking about stealing her money.

3. A 37-year-old female who previously held a managerial position in a large financial firm is brought to hospital by her

parents. According to the parents, the patient has not been coping with her work for the last few years and has gradually become withdrawn. She was fired from her work 3 years ago and since then, has been doing nothing but smoking in her bed all day. On mental state examination, her affect is blunted and she appears to have no motivation.

4. A 25-year-old male is brought to hospital as he was found to be trashing his apartment and throwing things from his window. He claims that everything in his flat is 'contaminated' and that voices are instructing him to get rid of all his possessions. He admits that this has been going on for a week. He agrees to a urine drug test, and the results are negative for all drugs. A week after admission, however, he makes a dramatic recovery and is now completely back to normal.

5. A 27-year-old male with no previous psychiatric history is brought to hospital by his family. His parents noticed that he has been 'high' for the last few months, and that his behaviour has become increasingly erratic. He was also noted to have strange beliefs, such as the world being flat and the government trying to prevent this fact from being disclosed. He even stated that he has a radio-transmitting device implanted in his head which allowed him to pick up the signals sent from space. His elated mood and strange beliefs continued for a year.

Psychotic illness II

A. Acute and transient psychotic disorder
B. Bipolar affective disorder
C. Catatonic schizophrenia
D. Hebephrenic schizophrenia
E. Paranoid schizophrenia
F. Residual schizophrenia
G. Schizoaffective disorder
H. Schizotypal disorder
I. Simple schizophrenia
J. Undifferentiated schizophrenia

The following patients present with a psychotic episode. Select the most appropriate diagnosis from the above that best fits with the following clinical description.

1. A 38-year-old male was previously in a general psychiatric ward for 2 years because he thought that the government was sending beams into his brain and trying to control his actions. He is now discharged into the community and seems less bothered by those thoughts. However, he prefers to stay indoors and does nothing all day, hardly socialising with anyone. On approaching him, he shows marked poverty of speech and a restricted affect.

2. A 46-year-old female is brought to hospital as she believes that she is a divine being in the process of transforming into God. She believes that she is able to control other people's feelings and behaviours. In the last few days, she has become increasingly aggressive to her neighbours as she thinks that they are stopping her from acquiring further powers. On examination, her speech is normal and no signs of elation or agitation are seen. Her psychiatric history is unremarkable.

3. A 38-year-old male is described as a 'loner' by his family as he does not seem to have any close friends. He usually spends his time alone at home because he becomes extremely anxious around other people. When talking to others, he feels that they are being nice to his face but that there's an alternative agenda. He likes to dress in silver clothing because he feels it brings him 'closer to cosmic forces'.

4. A 25-year-old male is taken to hospital by the police as he was found screaming on the streets. He had been trying to light himself with a lighter, claiming that he was invincible and had the power to fix all evil in the world. His speech was highly pressured and he complains that his thoughts are going out of control. According to hospital records, he had been admitted to hospital three times in the last year for similar episodes.

5. A 30-year-old male is brought to hospital by his family because of increasing concerns about his behaviour. In the last few months, the patient has been going through periods when his mind appears to be preoccupied, staring in space and maintaining a funny posture like a statue. On examination, he is mute and does not respond to any stimuli. His urine drug screen is negative.

The anxious patient

A. Adjustment disorder
B. Agoraphobia
C. Conversion disorder
D. Generalised anxiety disorder
E. Hypochondriasis
F. Obsessive-compulsive disorder
G. Panic disorder
H. Post-traumatic stress disorder
I. Social phobia
J. Somatisation

The following patients present with symptoms of anxiety. Select the most appropriate diagnosis from the above that best fits with the following clinical descriptions.

1. A 20-year-old male becomes anxious in the company of unfamiliar people and fears possible scrutiny by others. He worries that he will act in a way that will be humiliating or embarrassing, and he attempts to avoid such situations. He realises that this has resulted in him failing to get promoted at work.

2. A 30-year-old female avoids travelling alone, using public transport, or being in crowded places as this makes her feel anxious. She feels that such situations make her feel unsafe. She eventually becomes housebound as she identifies her home as being the only safe place for her.

3. A 32-year-old male has recurrent and persistent thoughts of contamination, which he recognises are irrational. He washes his hands repeatedly throughout the day, which relieves his anxiety. He also performs a ritual which must be performed in the correct order in order to prevent something dreadful happening to his wife.

4. A 37-year-old female, who previously held a managerial position in a large financial firm, presents to the clinic saying that she is no longer able to continue with her job. About a month ago, she started having episodes of dizziness and palpitations, coupled with the thought that she was 'going to die'. These

episodes only last for a few minutes, and seem to occur randomly at home, work, or outside. Although she is able to function normally between these episodes, she is now worried as to when these attacks will next come on.

5. A 22-year-old male is preoccupied with the fear that he has cancer. He has had a number of investigations which have not revealed any abnormalities, but is not reassured. He has visited three hospitals in the last year.

The stressful patient

A. Abnormal grief reaction
B. Acute stress reaction
C. Adjustment disorder
D. Agoraphobia
E. Conversion disorder
F. Depressive disorder
G. Generalised anxiety disorder
H. Normal grief reaction
I. Post-traumatic stress disorder
J. Simple (specific) phobia

The following patients present with a reaction to stress. Select the most appropriate diagnosis from the above that best fits with the following clinical descriptions.

1. A 65-year-old male was admitted to a medical ward with a history of chest pain, low mood, and weight loss. No medical cause was found. He said that about 12 days ago, his house was burgled and he lost his belongings. He progressed well in the ward and appeared cheerful, but as his discharge date approached, he complained of feeling 'not right' and refused to go back home.

2. A 47-year-old female and her son were involved in a car accident while she was driving. Her son unfortunately died in the accident, and she spent 2 weeks in hospital for a head injury. Although she made an uneventful recovery, 4 months after the accident, she started experiencing intrusive thoughts about the accident. She has been unable to get into a car and has avoided visiting the accident site. She complains of poor concentration, anxiety, and low mood.

3. A 22-year-old college student found out that her previously well father was killed in a car accident unexpectedly. She returns home and prepares for her father's funeral, but finds it very difficult. She is tearful, agitated, and unable to concentrate. Two years later, she is still mourning her father's death and has dropped out of college. She has avoided visiting the site of the accident, and also seems to deny the incident. Her father's room is left untouched since the day of the accident, and she pretends that he is still alive.

4. A 24-year-old medical student travels abroad for his elective. While going back to his residence late at night, he is held to a gunpoint by two masked figures asking for his money. He promptly hands his wallet and the assailants run away. He returns home but upon arrival, he feels numb and becomes tearful. The following day, he has recollections of the events but is no longer troubled by it.

5. A 32-year-old female is unable to walk following her sudden separation from her husband. She is now unable to walk unaided and requires a wheelchair, and her husband had agreed to visit her once a week to help her out. Neurological examination is inconsistent with her symptoms and investigations are all normal.

The patient with unexplained symptoms

A. Dissociative amnesia
B. Dissociative motor disease
C. Dysmorphophobia
D. Factitious disorder
E. Ganser's syndrome
F. Hypochondriasis
G. Malingering
H. Schizophrenia
I. Somatisation disorder
J. Trance and possession disorder

Select the most appropriate diagnosis from the above that fits with the following clinical descriptions.

1. A 23-year-old female presents to hospital complaining of abdominal pain. She was admitted to the surgical ward, but was very demanding of the nurses' attention. She underwent several blood tests and a colonoscopy, all of which were unremarkable. Once her investigations were completed, she self-discharged. Her records indicated that this was her fifth admission in 5 months, each admission resulting in self-discharge.

2. A 23-year-old female presents to hospital complaining of abdominal pain. She was waiting calmly and smiling, but when seen by the doctor, she starts screaming that she is in pain and demands that she be treated with morphine to alleviate the pain. However, her history and physical examination were inconsistent and investigations, including an X-ray, were unremarkable. A member of staff recognises her from a few weeks ago when she gave a different alias and demanded for morphine. He suspects that she is a heroin addict.

3. A 23-year-old female presents to hospital complaining of abdominal pain. While waiting in the emergency department, the ward staff retrieves her records and finds that she has been presenting almost on a weekly basis for the last 15 months with problems such as abdominal pain, headache, and constipation. On contacting her general practitioner, he informs that the patient presents on a weekly basis to his practice with minor

problems such as itches, dizziness, and joint aches. He further informs that she has been having difficulties with her partner for the last 2 years following their arranged marriage.

4. A 23-year-old female presents to hospital complaining of abdominal pain. While waiting to be seen, she demands that she be referred to the surgical team for further investigations, as she is highly anxious that she has colon cancer. She is eventually admitted and undergoes a colonoscopy, which was unremarkable. Despite reassurance from the surgeons, she is convinced that she has colon cancer as she feels that the surgeons are trying to be nice and are hiding the 'horrible facts' from her.

5. A 23-year-old female presents to hospital complaining of abdominal pain. While waiting to be seen, she is noted to have heavy vaginal bleeding. She was referred to the gynaecologists, who find that she had 'retained products of conception' in her uterus. On questioning, she denied any pregnancy but her husband informs that she had a miscarriage the day before. Otherwise, the patient's cognition is intact with a score of 30/30 on the mini-mental state examination.

The patient with memory problems

A. Anterograde amnesia
B. Confabulation
C. Deja vu
D. Delusional memory
E. Delusional misidentification
F. Dissociative amnesia
G. Dissociative fugue
H. Jamais vu
I. Malingering
J. No mental illness

The following patients present with memory problems. Select the most appropriate item from the above that best matches the clinical description.

1. A 56-year-old male suffering from schizophrenia is discharged home as his mental state is now stable after a 4-week admission. On returning home with the social worker, however, he initially says that his house seemed unfamiliar, as if it was like a stranger's house, but he quickly recognises it as his own.

2. A 45-year-old male with a history of alcohol abuse is admitted to a ward. He was oriented to the ward but is unable to remember the name of the ward or hospital. He is also unable to remember the name of his primary nurse despite seeing her everyday. His psychiatrist comes and interviews him, but he repeatedly asks her name.

3. A 24-year-old female recently lost her fiancé in a car crash. Following this, she is reported missing by her family as they are unable to get hold of her, but police reports indicate that she was working in a bar abroad. Four weeks later, she returns home in a completely fit state but is unable to recall where she has been.

4. A 40-year-old female suffering from schizophrenia breaks down into tears during the ward round, saying that she was raped by her brothers during childhood. Collateral history from her mother indicates that she is the only child, but she remains

adamant that her brothers raped her. She points to stretch marks on her abdomen and says that they are proofs of the sexual assault.

5. A 43-year-old male had an argument with his wife, as he was not forthcoming about where he has been spending his time during the day. When the wife confronts him whether he was out gambling, he replies: 'Yes yes, I have been gambling ... in fact I won quite a bit!' However, his explanations are unreliable and appear to change significantly during the conversation depending on what the wife says. He has a history of alcohol abuse.

Mood disorders I

A. Bipolar affective disorder
B. Cyclothymia
C. Depressive episode, mild
D. Depressive episode, moderate
E. Depressive episode, severe
F. Dysthymia
G. Hypermania
H. Hypomania
I. Mania
J. Recurrent depressive disorder

The following patients present with mood disturbances. Select the most appropriate diagnosis from the above that best fits with the given clinical descriptions.

1. A 28-year-old female presents to the clinic complaining of low mood. She explains that she has always felt low, as if something was missing from her heart. Other than that, she has no complaints, and her sleep and appetite are both healthy. She is able to keep her job and appears to be enjoying a reasonable social life.

2. A 28-year-old female presents to the clinic complaining of low mood. She has been feeling like this for the last 3 months and is unable to identify any triggers. She feels tearful and does not seem to enjoy things she once did. She is still able to go to work, although at times it has been difficult for her to concentrate. Her appetite has decreased but she manages to sleep around 7 hours per night. Her past psychiatric history is unremarkable.

3. A 28-year-old female presents to the clinic complaining of low mood. She describes her mood as 'depressing' and is unable to do anything. Because of her low mood, she has not eaten for 3 days. She mentions that a year ago, she was feeling on top of the world and went through periods when she did not have to sleep. On that occasion, she was admitted to hospital because her parents thought that she was going 'out of control'.

4. A 28-year-old female presents to the clinic, but she is overactive and unable to sit still. When she finally starts talking, she

is clearly over-excited and her thoughts are hard to follow. She vaguely mentions about having a special connection with God, and that she is the 'chosen one'. She believes that she has the power to heal all human suffering from the world, and even claims that she is hearing God's voice at present. Her past psychiatric history is unremarkable.

5. A 28-year-old female presents to the clinic, but the doctor is unable to fully carry out an assessment as the patient is mute and does not make any eye contact. According to the mother, the patient has been like this for the last few weeks and has hardly eaten anything. She has told her mother that she is 'dead' and thus does not need to be fed. Earlier today, she was found stacking a pile of wood in the garden as she wanted to cremate her dead body. Her past psychiatric history is unremarkable.

Mood disorders II

A. Atypical depression
B. Bonding failure
C. Childhood depression
D. Depression in the elderly
E. Dysthymia
F. Postpartum blues
G. Postpartum depression
H. Postpartum psychosis
I. Premenstrual syndrome
J. Seasonal affective disorder

Select the most appropriate diagnosis from the above for each of the following statements.

1. Depressive episode whereby the patient complains of depressed mood less often and instead complains of physical symptoms such as disturbed sleep and somatic problems. These patients remain at substantially higher risk of completed suicide.

2. Affective episode temporally related to childbirth with an abrupt onset at about 2–4 weeks. The episodes may be marked with psychotic features such as hallucinations and delusions relating to the baby. Risk is increased in first time mothers and instrumental deliveries.

3. Depressive episode in which the patient does complain of low mood, but appears to lack the biological and other associated features of depression. The patient can present with features such as hypersomnia, hyperphagia, and heaviness of limbs.

4. Clinical symptoms involve low mood, hypersomnia, fatigue, increased appetite, and weight gain. Social functioning can be decreased during the duration of the episode. The episodes follow a recurring pattern, and light therapy is a suggested form of treatment.

5. Depressive episode characterised by low mood, anhedonia, and altered sleep and appetite. In addition, it may manifest with somatisation, behavioural disruptions, and substance abuse. Male to female rate is roughly equal, and completed suicide is rare.

Personality disorders I

A. Anankastic
B. Anxious (avoidant)
C. Dependent
D. Dissocial
E. Emotionally unstable – borderline
F. Emotionally unstable – impulsive
G. Histrionic
H. Paranoid
I. Passive aggressive
J. Schizoid

Select the most appropriate diagnosis from the above that fits with the following clinical descriptions.

1. A 45-year-old male works in data processing from home. He has never had a relationship, and was often described as a loner at school. He hardly has any friends, but is not bothered by it as he prefers working and living at home alone.

2. A 30-year-old female works as a medical secretary. She always arrives to work 2 hours before everyone else as she likes to ensure that her desk and the office is in order. She usually leaves work 2 hours late as she has difficulty completing her work on time due to her thorough checking and rechecking. The other secretaries think she is stubborn and become annoyed with her when she insists that they do things in a similar way.

3. A 50-year-old female describes herself as 'always having mood swings'. She goes out on a blind date with a man she has met over the Internet, but while having a conversation about politics in a restaurant, she gets upset about a comment her date makes. She starts screaming at him and throws dishes on the floor, screaming: 'Look what you made me do.'

4. A 22-year-old bubbly female college student has a lot of friends, but they often complain that she has verbal diarrhoea and finds her to be too dominating in conversations. She often wears very short skirts and likes being the centre of attention. While out clubbing, she trips over and scratches her leg but the following day, she tells her friends that she was attacked in the club and had to go to the hospital to have her leg treated.

5. An 18-year-old student who recently started university finds it hard to talk to others. He would like to make new friends, but finds everything too intimidating. He rationalises that he would not fit in as he comes from another part of the country and thus would have nothing in common. Because he is scared of being rejected by his classmates, rather than attending classes, he spends the majority of the time alone in the library and at home.

Personality disorders II

A. Antisocial
B. Avoidant
C. Borderline
D. Dependent
E. Histrionic
F. Narcissistic
G. Obsessive compulsive
H. Paranoid
I. Schizoid
J. Schizotypal

Select the most appropriate diagnosis from the above that fits with the following clinical descriptions.

1. A 22-year-old male gets angry after finding out that he failed his college examinations, saying that the paper was badly set. He has very few friends as he is very picky and feels some of his peers are not up to his level. His parents aren't too worried, saying that 'he has always been like that.'

2. A 20-year-old female with a history of childhood sexual abuse has chronic suicidal ideation. She is currently in an abusive relationship marked by arguments, but still prefers to be with her boyfriend. She presents to the hospital today for deliberate self-harm, and tells the duty doctor: 'You are the best doctor I have ever come across'.

3. A 29-year-old female, who has always been described as odd and strange by her friends, has a very strong interest in the occult and mystics, and believes that she is able to see spirits. Despite coming from a middle class English family, she prefers to wear traditional Native American clothing as she believes this will help her connect with nature better. She once saw a cat being run over by a car, and decided to become a vegetarian then as she took the incident as being a divine message from God.

4. A 19-year-old male dropped out of school at the age of 13 years for violent behaviour. He has been spending his days doing nothing but pacing around the streets and pick-pocketing from

strangers. He has been convicted several times in the past for armed robbery, and claims that this was done for self-defence. He appears to have no remorse for the victims, and has never been able to maintain a relationship.

5. A 29-year-old waitress has never been able to live alone. Ever since finishing university, she has always lived in an apartment with her friends as she finds the prospect of living alone too daunting. She constantly needs reassurances and support from her friends, and does not appear to be able to make up her own mind about anything. When her friends ask her for a favour, she always complies as she finds it difficult to refuse them.

The patient with unusual eating habits

A. Anorexia nervosa
B. Binge eating disorder
C. Bipolar affective disorder
D. Bulimia nervosa
E. Depression
F. Diabetes mellitus
G. Obsessive-compulsive disorder
H. Paranoid schizophrenia
I. Specific phobia
J. No mental illness

The following patients present with unusual eating patterns. Select the appropriate item from the above that is the most likely underlying diagnosis in the following scenarios.

1. A 21-year-old female has not been eating adequately for the last 6 months and has lost approximately 15 kg in weight. She claims that all food and tap water are contaminated with cyanide and thus has been taking food supplements and bottled water only. On examination, her BMI is 15 and she has not had her menstrual periods for almost 3 months.

2. A 20-year-old male spends the majority of his time at home eating greasy fast food, playing on the computer, and sleeping all day. He does not seem to engage in any physical activities despite constant encouragement from his family, citing that he is 'too lazy'. On examination, his BMI is 34 and abdominal stretch marks are noted.

3. A 28-year-old female is brought to hospital by her family as she has lost a considerable amount of weight in 4 weeks. She describes having no appetite or energy, and has lost interest in looking after herself. This seems to have started following her divorce, and she feels guilty about the break up of her marriage all the time. Her BMI is 19.

4. A 19-year-old female is brought to hospital as she collapsed at work. She reports that she is in the midst of a 'strict dieting regimen' as she feels that she is too fat. For the last 8 months, she

has been eating a small portion of salad a day, working out 5 days a week, and taking appetite suppressants. She has not had a menstrual cycle in 3 months. On examination, she is weak, anaemic, and her BMI is 16.

5. A 21-year-old female is complaining of feeling bad about herself because she feels that everyone around her is looking down on her. As a means of releasing her stress, she goes through periods of frantically eating three boxes of cereals and eight bars of chocolates in one go. Following this, she feels even worse and ends up making herself sick. Her BMI is 25 and her history is significant for polysubstance and alcohol use.

Physical consequences of eating disorders

A. Arrhythmia and cardiomyopathy
B. Cerebral atrophy (pseudoatrophy)
C. Tachycardia and malignant hypertension
D. Hypernatraemia and hyperkalaemia
E. Hypoglycaemia with raised cholesterol and amylase
F. Hypophosphataemia
G. Hypothalamic dysfunction with decreased gonadotrophins
H. Lanugo hair
I. Metabolic acidosis
J. Russell's sign

Select the most appropriate item from the above for each of the following statements.

1. Included in the ICD-10 diagnostic criteria for anorexia.

2. Consequence of excessive laxative use.

3. Leading cause of mortality in patients with anorexia.

4. Indicative of repeated self-induced vomiting.

5. Core feature of refeeding syndrome.

Answers

Psychotic illness I

1. **D.** Hebephrenic schizophrenia is a subtype of schizophrenia that is characterised by changes in affect (flattening or incongruity of affect), thought disorder, and behaviour that is aimless or disjointed. Mannerisms are also quite common. Hallucinations and delusions are usually fragmentary and do not dominate the clinical picture. Individuals tend to become socially isolated and tend to develop prominent negative symptoms. This type of schizophrenia is usually diagnosed in adolescents or young people.

2. **E.** Paranoid schizophrenia is a common subtype of schizophrenia where delusions and hallucinations are prominent. The delusions are not necessarily persecutory in nature, but they all must pertain to the individual, whether it be grandiose, love, etc. Other symptoms such as abnormalities of affect, catatonic symptoms, or thought disorder may be present but not to a significant degree.

3. **I.** Simple schizophrenia is an uncommon and controversial subtype of schizophrenia, which is characterised by at least a 1 year history of progressive development of negative symptoms (apathy, blunting of affect, lack of initiative and drive), gradual changes in social behaviour, and social withdrawal. There is no evidence of preceding acute psychotic symptoms.

4. **A.** Acute and transient psychotic disorder is characterised by the acute onset of psychotic symptoms, usually within 2 weeks. The symptoms resolve within a few weeks and in some cases after a few days. It is best thought of as a 'one-off' psychotic episode.

5. **G.** Schizoaffective disorder comprises symptoms that meet some diagnostic criteria for both an affective disorder (depression, mania, mixed type) and schizophrenia. The symptoms must occur simultaneously and in approximately equal proportions. It does *not* include patients with schizophrenia who go on to develop affective symptoms or patients with an affective disorder who go on to develop psychotic symptoms.

Notes

- For an ICD-10 diagnosis of schizophrenia, one of the following must be fulfilled for at least 1 month:
  - At least *one* of the following must be present: thought insertion, withdrawal, broadcast, echo; voices giving a running commentary or discussing the patient's behaviour; delusional perception; passivity phenomena, delusion of control; persistent delusions. These are mostly Schneider's first-rank symptoms.
  - At least *two* of the following must be present: persistent hallucinations in any modality; formal thought disorder (such as incoherent speech and neologisms); catatonic symptoms; negative symptoms; decrease in social functioning.

- For a DSM-IV diagnosis at least two symptoms (delusions, hallucinations, disorganised speech, negative symptoms, catatonic symptoms) must be present for at least 1 month, including signs of disturbance for at least 6 months.

Psychotic illness II

1. **F.** Residual schizophrenia is a chronic stage in schizophrenic illnesses where there is a clear progression from an active psychotic phase to a chronic negative phase. The negative phase comprises of psychomotor retardation, affective blunting, reduced motivation, reduced speech output, and a decline in social functioning. Both simple and residual schizophrenia are similar in that they are marked by a negative phase, but residual schizophrenia is always preceded by an active psychotic phase while simple schizophrenia does not.

2. **E.** Paranoid schizophrenia is marked by hallucinations and delusions. The delusions are usually paranoid in that they relate to the patient, but it does not necessarily have to be persecutory in nature. In this example, the patient is experiencing delusions of grandiosity with some persecution. Grandiose delusions are commonly seen in bipolar affective disorder, but this has been ruled out in this patient due to lack of manic symptoms.

3. **H.** Schizotypal disorder is classified as a schizophrenic illness in ICD-10, but belongs to personality disorder in DSM-IV. It is thought to be related to schizophrenia in that the incidence is higher in relatives of patients with schizophrenia. It is similar

to schizophrenia but lacks the hallucinations and delusions (although transient psychotic experiences may occur). Characteristics seen are ideas of references, odd beliefs, eccentric appearance and speech, inappropriate affect, suspiciousness, and social anxiety.

4. B. Bipolar affective disorder is a mood disorder characterised by the presence of several depressive and manic/hypomanic episodes during the lifetime of a patient. In this example, the patient is exhibiting grandiose delusions with manic symptoms such as pressured speech and flight of ideas.

5. C. Catatonic schizophrenia is dominated by psychomotor disturbances, which may fluctuate between extremes of excitement and hyperkinesis to stupor and mutism. Catatonic behaviours such as automatic obedience and posturing are also seen.

Notes
- Undifferentiated schizophrenia is a condition that meets the general diagnostic criteria for schizophrenia, but does not fit with one particular subtype. For example, a patient may exhibit thought withdrawal but have no other behavioural symptoms to specify the type of schizophrenia.

The anxious patient

1. I. Social phobia is characterised by a marked fear of being the focus of attention and the fear that one will behave in an embarrassing or humiliating way. This leads to avoidance of social situations such as speaking or eating in public. The individual may present with blushing, shaking, nausea, vomiting, or urgency of micturition during these situations.

2. B. Agoraphobia is the fear and avoidance of crowded places, public places (such as shops), travelling alone (e.g. on trains or buses), and being away from home. There are symptoms of anxiety, which are restricted to these 'unsafe' situations only. Agoraphobia may or may not be associated with panic attacks.

3. F. Obsessive-compulsive disorder is characterised by recurrent obsessional thoughts and compulsions. Obsessions are recurrent and unpleasant thoughts, images, or impulses that intrude into the patient's mind and are recognised by the patient as being his or her own thoughts. Compulsions are acts that are repeated constantly and carried out to relieve anxiety or to prevent an event from happening, such as a loved one getting hurt. The patient attempts to resist these obsessions and compulsions, often with limited success, and recognises that they are irrational or absurd. The obsessions and compulsions cause significant social and occupational distress.

4. **G.** Panic disorder is characterised by recurrent panic attacks. An episode of a panic attack develops rapidly and peaks at around 10 minutes, and usually does not last for more than 20–30 minutes. Typical symptoms include palpitations, sweating, trembling, chest pain, shortness of breath, numbness or tingling, fear of losing control, and a fear of dying. It is important to exclude a substance misuse disorder or a medical disorder such as hyperthyroidism, Cushing's syndrome, hypoglycaemia, phaeochromocytoma, anaemia, and cardiac arrhythmias. Comorbidity with other psychiatric disorders is common (agoraphobia, depression, and other anxiety disorders).

5. **E.** Hypochondriasis is the persistent preoccupation of having a serious physical disorder or the preoccupation with a presumed deformity or disfigurement (body dysmorphic disorder). The symptoms cause distress and lead the patient to seek medical treatment or investigations, but there is a refusal to accept reassurance.

Notes

- Generalised anxiety disorder is characterised by generalised, persistent anxiety or excessive worry about daily events and problems, associated with muscle tension, sleep disturbance, and autonomic hyperactivity. This is a chronic disorder lasting longer than 6 months.

- Anxiety disorders can be simplified as follows:
  - Is anxiety generalised or episodic? If general: *generalised anxiety.*
  - If episodic, is the trigger known or random? If random: *panic disorder.*

– If trigger known, specify trigger as:
Simple phobia (objects or situations)
Agoraphobia (unsafe places)
Social phobia (social situations).

The stressful patient

1. **C.** An adjustment disorder must occur within 1 month of a psychosocial stressor and should not occur for longer than 6 months, except in the case of a prolonged depressive reaction, which may last up to 2 years (ICD-10). Symptoms cause significant distress but are not severe enough to meet the criteria of a major psychiatric illness such as depression. A bereavement or grief reaction also fits into this category.

2. **I.** Post-traumatic stress disorder is a severe psychological disturbance that occurs following a traumatic event. Symptoms (ICD-10) include persistent reliving of the incident in the form of flashbacks or nightmares, avoidance of situations resembling or associated with the incident, inability to recall completely or partially some aspects of the event, and persistent symptoms of arousal (difficulty concentrating, irritability, difficulty falling asleep, hypervigilance, and exaggerated startle response).

3. **A.** Abnormal grief reaction is grief that is delayed (by more than 2 weeks), prolonged (greater than 6 months), or abnormal in grief content. Symptoms include feelings of worthlessness, excessive guilt, suicidal ideation, hallucinatory experiences (other than the voice or image of the deceased), and denial. On the other hand, normal grief is characterised by disbelief, numbness, anger, sadness, tearfulness, and pseudohallucinations of the deceased, which eventually resolves by 6 months.

4. **B.** An acute stress reaction is a transient disorder that usually develops within an hour of a stressor and resolves within a few hours or days. Symptoms may include disorientation, feeling 'dazed', aggression, social withdrawal, anger, and despair.

5. **E.** Conversion or dissociative disorders are associated with a loss or disturbance of normal functioning. The symptoms develop in close relationship to a psychological stressor. Symptoms include paralysis, sensory loss, seizures, amnesia, and loss of speech.

The disturbance conforms to the patient's understanding of the disorder and physical examination is often inconsistent with the patient's symptoms. Investigations are normal. Most symptoms resolve after a few weeks or months, but some disorders may become chronic if associated with insoluble or unbearable personal problems. In this vignette, the patient displays dissociative motor disorder.

Notes
- Simple (specific) phobia refers to an intense fear induced by the presence of a specific object or situation, such as heights and spiders.

The patient with unexplained symptoms

1. **D.** In factitious disorder, patients falsify symptoms of medical or psychiatric illnesses for the purpose of receiving medical attention and treatment. The motives for such behaviour are usually unclear. It is also known as Munchausen's syndrome.

2. **G.** Malingering is the falsification of symptoms for secondary gain. This may include attempting to escape a prison sentence, military service, or an attempt to obtain an opiate prescription.

3. **I.** In somatisation disorder, the individual is preoccupied with *physical symptoms* for which no medical cause has been found. It causes significant distress and functional impairment. The patient often has a history of consulting many doctors for an opinion and is not reassured by normal investigation results. Management involves acknowledging the severity of the symptoms and distress, minimising further investigations, ensuring that one doctor co-ordinates future care, and exploration of symptoms in the context of personal and emotional meaning. Cognitive behavioural therapy (CBT) and psychotherapy may be helpful.

4. **F.** In hypochondriasis, the patient is preoccupied with the fear of having a serious *medical illness* such as cancer and is not reassured by negative investigations. The patient constantly seeks medical advice and reassurance. There may be a history of childhood or parental illness or abnormal illness behaviour.

It is distinguished from somatisation disorder where the pre-occupation is with symptoms.

5. **A.** Dissociative amnesia is memory loss that exceeds one's forgetfulness, and can be selective. It involves inability to recall part of one's identity or life. It occurs in clear consciousness and short-term memory (retention) is usually normal. It is a subtype of dissociative/conversion disorder. The signs and symptoms do not conform to medical knowledge and are often based on the patient's own understanding.

Notes

• Ganser's syndrome is a dissociative disorder with four central features: psychogenic physical symptoms, approximate answers, pseudohallucinations, and clouding of consciousness. On questioning, patients give inconsistent answers and may present with amnesia for the whole episode.

• Trance and possession disorder is characterised with trance (temporary alteration of the state of consciousness, including loss of personal identity, awareness of surroundings, and limitation of movements) and possession (conviction that the individual has been possessed or taken over by another being). These must be unwanted and occurring outside religious or culturally accepted situations.

• Dysmorphophobia is a condition whereby the individual feels that a part of his or her body is disfigured or out of proportion, and experiences great anxiety and distress as a result of this preoccupation. These beliefs are overvalued ideas or obsessions, but not delusional in intensity. In ICD-10 it is classified under hypochondriacal disorder.

The patient with memory problems

1. **H.** Jamais vu is the experience of a situation being unfamiliar even though it has been experienced before. It can be a normal experience but may also occur in some disorders such as temporal lobe epilepsy and schizophrenia. The opposite of jamais vu is déjà vu, where an experience is perceived as being familiar although objectively it has never been experienced before.

2. **A.** The patient in the scenario is suffering from Korsakoff's syndrome, a recognised complication of chronic alcohol abuse. The prominent feature here is that of anterograde amnesia, which is the inability to form new memories. The converse of this is retrograde amnesia, which is the inability to recall memory before an amnesic episode.

3. **G.** Dissociative fugue is associated with a stressful event and involves the individual undertaking an unexpected but organised journey from home during which self-care is maintained. The patient's behaviour may appear completely normal to passers by. There is partial or complete amnesia for the event.
   - Dissociative amnesia refers to memory loss that may be selective and is a possible choice. However, the vignette describes the patient taking a trip with evidence of adequate self-care, and thus dissociative fugue would be the better answer.

4. **D.** Delusional memory is used to describe either a situation where a patient 'remembers' past experiences that clearly did not occur, or when a normal memory is given a delusional meaning. The vignette described here refers to the first definition, as the patient claims she remembers an event that did not happen.

5. **B.** Confabulation is the falsification of memory occurring in clear consciousness in association with organic amnesia. In these cases, patients fill the conversation with anything that comes to mind in an effort to mask their memory loss and thus the content is heavily influenced by the conversation taking place. Confabulation is often seen in patients with Korsakoff's syndrome.

Notes
- Delusional misidentification refers to patients being unable to correctly identify another person or place correctly, for example claiming that an individual has been replaced by an imposter.

- Malingering refers to the conscious production of false symptoms for clear secondary gain and memory loss may be faked for clear gain, such as an individual trying to avoid a court hearing by claiming to have lost all memory.

Mood disorders I

1. **F.** Dysthymia is characterised by the presence of chronic low mood, which must be present for at least 2 years but not severe enough for a diagnosis of a depressive disorder. There may be intervening periods of normal mood but these do not last longer than a few weeks.

2. **C.** Depressive disorders are classified into mild, moderate, severe without psychotic features, and severe with psychotic features according to ICD-10. The severity of the episode is dependent on the number and intensity of the depressive symptoms, and must be present for at least 2 weeks:
   - *Core* depressive symptoms are low mood, decreased energy, anhedonia.
   - *Associated* symptoms are disturbed sleep, diminished appetite, self-harm impulses, disturbed attention/concentration, feelings of guilt/worthlessness, hopelessness, low self-esteem.
   The following are the diagnostic guidelines for ICD-10:
   - *Mild*: Total of four core and associated (at least two core symptoms).
   - *Moderate*: Six core and associated symptoms (at least two core symptoms).
   - *Severe*: Eight core and associated symptoms (all core symptoms needed).
   A diagnosis of *recurrent depressive disorder* is made when a patient has at least two depressive disorders without any previous history of hypomania or mania.

3. **A.** The vignette described sounds like a mild or moderate depressive episode, but given the patient's previous history of a manic episode, the best diagnosis is bipolar affective disorder, which by definition is characterised by two or more episodes of significant mood disturbance, of which one episode must be hypomania or mania.
   - Bipolar affective disorder is further subdivided into two. Type I is characterised by depressive episodes with at least one *manic episode*, while type II is characterised by depressive episodes with at least one *hypomanic episode* (but not mania).

4. **I.** Mania is an episode characterised by symptoms of elevated mood (for at least 1 week), increased activity, pressure of

speech, flight of ideas, decreased need for sleep, loss of social inhibitions, and reckless behaviour (overspending, reckless driving). There may be mood-congruent psychotic symptoms, which frequently are grandiose delusions and second-person auditory hallucinations.

• Hypomania is a milder form of mania, in which the patient clearly has an elevated mood but the symptoms are not severe enough to cause disruption to social life.

• The vignette described here cannot be bipolar affective disorder because this was the first affective episode for the patient.

5. E. The vignette describes an episode of severe depression characterised with psychotic features. Psychotic symptoms are mood congruent and include delusions of guilt, worthlessness, poverty, nihilistic delusions, and second-person auditory hallucinations of voices that are derogatory in nature.

Notes
• Hypermania does not exist.

• Cyclothymia is a persistent instability of mood characterised by mild depression and mild elation, none of which are severe enough to qualify for a formal diagnosis of bipolar affective disorder or recurrent depressive disorder.

Mood disorders II
1. D. Depression in the elderly is more likely to present with somatic, anxiety, or hypochondriacal symptoms, nihilistic delusions, delusions of poverty or physical illness, cognitive impairment (pseudodementia), and severe psychomotor agitation or retardation. Pseudodementia is poor concentration and memory associated with depression that can mimic dementia. It usually improves when the symptoms of depression resolve.

2. H. Postpartum (puerperal) psychosis occurs in 0.2% of live births. Features include labile mood, perplexity, disorientation, insomnia, psychotic symptoms, and thoughts of suicide or harming the baby. Other risk factors include lack of social support and a personal or family history of postpartum psychosis, bipolar affective disorder, or schizophrenia.

3. A. Features of atypical depression include a reactive mood, reversal of diurnal variation in mood (mood better in the morning), increased appetite, weight gain, and increased sleep. Atypical depression is thought to respond better to monoamine oxidase inhibitors.

4. J. Seasonal affective disorder is associated with recurrent episodes of depression, which has a seasonal pattern of episodes in winter. Mild hypomania may occur in the summer. Ultraviolet light therapy is associated with a good response.

5. C. In young children depression may present as irritability, hyperactivity, tantrums, apathy, poor feeding, somatisation, and regression (enuresis, soiling). In older children features include school refusal, poor performance at school, somatisation, and poor sleep. The prevalence of depression before puberty is roughly equal between the sexes but increases in females after puberty.

Notes

- Postpartum blues ('baby blues') is experienced by up to 75% of mothers and occurs about 2–3 days after birth and lasts for 1–2 days. The mother is typically tearful and emotionally labile, but this is self-limiting and only reassurance is usually required.

- Postpartum depression is a significant depressive episode that occurs in 10–15% of pregnant women, peaking around 3–4 weeks after childbirth. The symptoms are similar to that of any other depressive episode, but usually are related to the baby's health or ability to cope. Risk factors are history of depression, single motherhood, ambivalence towards the pregnancy, and poor social support.

- Bonding failure occurs when the mother fails to develop a normal loving, emotional relationship with her baby, usually in the context of unwanted, ambivalent pregnancies or depressive illness.

- Premenstrual syndrome is a collection of psychological (mood disturbance, insomnia, poor concentration) and physical (headache, bloating) symptoms occurring 24 hours after ovulation, and quickly relieved by menstrual flow.

Personality disorders I

Personality disorders are deeply ingrained and enduring patterns of behaviour, which manifest as inflexible responses to a broad range of personal and social situations, and are a significant deviation from how the average person in a given culture thinks, feels, and relates to others. They are frequently associated with subjective distress and problems in social functioning.

1. **J.** Schizoid personality disorder is characterised by emotional coldness and detachment, preference for solitary activities, excessive introspection, no desire for relationships, indifference to either praise or criticism, and a marked insensitivity to social norms and conventions (but this is unintentional). These patients are 'loners' who prefer their own company.

2. **A.** Anankastic (or obsessive) personality is characterised by excessive concern with details and order, excessive conscientiousness, perfectionism that interferes with task completion, feelings of excessive doubt and caution, rigidity and stubbornness, and insistence that others submit to his or her way of doing things.

3. **F.** Emotionally unstable personality disorder has two subtypes. The impulsive subtype is associated with a tendency to act unexpectedly without consideration of the consequences, quarrelsome behaviour, outbursts of anger or violence, and an inability to control such behavioural explosions. Unstable mood and difficulty in maintaining a course of action that offers no immediate reward are also seen.

4. **G.** Histrionic personality disorder is characterised by a shallow and labile affect, over dramatisation or exaggerated expression of emotions, suggestibility (easily influenced by others), over concern with physical appearance, inappropriate seductiveness in appearance and behaviour, and the need to be the centre of attention.

5. **B.** Anxious personality disorder is characterised by persistent feelings of tension and apprehension, the belief that one is socially inferior, and excessive preoccupation with being criticised or rejected. This leads to avoidance of social and

occupational activities and unwillingness to engage with people unless certain of being liked. Unlike those with schizoid personality disorder, these patients want social interaction but are unable to do so.

Notes

• The types of personality disorders differ slightly between ICD-10 and DSM-IV, and those listed in this question derive from ICD-10. Dissocial personality disorder is known as antisocial in DSM-IV, and emotionally unstable impulsive type does not exist in DSM-IV.

• Passive aggressive is also known as negativistic personality disorder and characterised by passive resistance to authoritarian circumstances, manifesting as procrastination, stubbornness, resentment, and forgetfulness. For example, a person who is opposed to a specific project may frequently miss meetings or make errors as a means of protest.

Personality disorders II

1. **F.** Narcissistic personality disorder includes a grandiose sense of self-importance, preoccupation with fantasies of unlimited success, the belief that he/she is special and should only associate with other special or high-status people, a sense of entitlement, the need for excessive admiration, a lack of empathy, and envy towards others or believes that others are envious of him/her.

2. **C.** Borderline personality disorder is characterised by disturbances in self-image and/or internal preferences (such as sexuality), intense and unstable relationships, self-harming, excessive efforts to avoid abandonment, and chronic feelings of emptiness. A fairly significant proportion of deliberate self-harmers presenting to hospital fall into this category.

3. **J.** Schizotypal disorder is classified as a personality disorder in DSM-IV but not in ICD-10 (schizophrenic spectrum disorder). Features include eccentric appearance or behaviour, cold and aloof affect, odd beliefs and magical thinking that is inconsistent with social norms, paranoid ideas, unusual perceptual experiences, and transient quasi-psychotic episodes.

4. A. Antisocial personality disorder is characterised by irresponsibility and disregard for social norms and rules, callous disregard for the feelings of others, tendency to become aggressive, inability to experience guilt, inability to learn from punishment, tendency to blame others, and an inability to maintain relationships.

5. D. Dependent personality disorder is characterised by the need of encouragement from others to make important decisions, inability to make everyday decisions without the need for excessive reassurance and advice from others, feelings of helplessness when left alone, undue compliance with the wishes of others, and an unwillingness to make even reasonable demands on the people one depends on.

Notes

- The choices in this question derive from the DSM-IV classification of personality disorders, which differ slightly from ICD-10. Passive-aggressive disorder was recognised as a personality disorder in the old DSM-III, but was omitted in DSM-IV and put in the appendix as there were controversies regarding its use.

- Paranoid personality is marked by a strong sense of suspiciousness, sensitivity to setbacks, tendency to bear grudges, and an unwillingness to forgive. Other features include a high sense of entitlement to personal rights, persistent self-referential attitudes, and a tendency to distort experiences as being hostile or threatening.

The patient with unusual eating habits

1. H. The patient in this vignette has decreased food intake associated with decreased weight and physical abnormalities, which all stems from her delusional beliefs regarding poisoned food and water. The presence of this delusion therefore suggests a diagnosis of schizophrenia.

2. J. The patient in this vignette is obese due to his BMI of 34 (obesity defined as BMI >30), but the underlying cause of this obesity is his unhealthy eating habits and physical inactivity. There is thus no evidence of a mental illness, but treatments should be mainly behavioural and psychological to re-establish sensible eating and physical activity.

3. E. Depression is the underlying cause of this patient's decreased appetite, as evidenced by her anergia, anhedonia, and constant sense of guilt.

4. A. The ICD-10 diagnostic criteria for anorexia nervosa are BMI of less than 17.5 (or body weight at least 15% less than expected), self-induced weight loss (such as avoidance of fattening foods), self-perception of being fat with fear of obesity, and endocrine dysfunction (such as amenorrhoea in women and impotence in males). The patient in this vignette fulfils these criteria and thus anorexia is the likely diagnosis.

5. D. The ICD-10 diagnostic criteria for bulimia nervosa are recurrent episodes of binge eating, persistent preoccupation with eating (craving), attempts to counteract the fattening effects of food through the use of compensatory mechanisms (such as self-induced vomiting, purging, use of appetite suppressants, excessive exercise), and the perception of being too fat with an intrusive dread of fatness. The usual age of onset is later than anorexia, and is usually in the region of late teens to 30 years old.

Notes

• Binge eating disorder is similar to bulimia nervosa, but is not associated with the compensatory vomiting or purging efforts.

• When assessing patients with low weight, it is always important to rule out an organic cause such as diabetes mellitus, malabsorption syndromes, and endocrine diseases (including Addisons and thyroid disorders).

• Poor prognostic factors for anorexia nervosa include longer illness duration, older age of onset, being male, poor parental relationship, and excessive weight loss. Anorexia nervosa usually has an onset around 13–20 years old, and has a male to female ratio of 1:10–20. It is seen more commonly in social classes I and II in industrialised countries, and is more frequent in specific occupations such as models and dancers.

• Efforts to lose weight are seen both in anorexia and bulimia, and vomiting is seen in both conditions.

- Treatment for both eating disorders are education, pharmacological (selective serotonin reuptake inhibitors such as fluoxetine), and psychological (CBT and family therapy). The UK NICE guidelines for anorexia recommend hospital treatment if one of the following criteria are met: BMI <13.5, severe electrolyte imbalance, cardiac complications, severe suicide risk, and failure of outpatient treatment.

Physical consequences of eating disorders

1. **G.** Endocrine complications resulting from disruption of the hypothalamic–pituitary–adrenal (HPA) axis is one of the diagnostic criteria for anorexia nervosa, and this commonly manifest as amenorrhea. Other endocrine disturbances seen in anorexia are raised growth hormone and cortisol levels.

2. **I.** Metabolic acidosis with hypokalaemia is seen with excessive use of laxatives, as bicarbonate and fluid are lost from the gut. There is also evidence that excessive laxative use can lead to renal tubular acidosis. On the other hand, metabolic alkalosis is seen with frequent vomiting, as hydrochloric acid is lost from the stomach.

3. **A.** Cardiovascular complications of anorexia nervosa account for 10% of mortality, and these include significant bradycardia, hypotension (systolic BP less than 70), arrhythmias, ECG changes (QT prolongation may occasionally lead to sudden death), and cardiomyopathies (also prolapsed mitral valve and decreased left ventricular mass).

4. **J.** Russell's sign refers to callused skin on the backs of hands (over the knuckles) due to repeated manual induction of vomiting. Other signs of repeated self-induced vomiting are parotid gland enlargement, eroded tooth enamel, and oesophageal tears.

5. **F.** Refeeding syndrome occurs when a previously starved or severely malnourished patient is recommenced on a normal diet. Upon being refed, carbohydrate metabolism and insulin secretion occur, leading to cellular uptake of phosphate. The resulting hypophosphataemia generally triggers non-specific symptoms, but these can lead to rhabdomyolysis, leucocyte dysfunction, respiratory failure, arrhythmias, coma, seizures,

and sometimes death. This phenomenon usually occurs within 4 days of refeeding and thus regular monitoring of kidney function and electrolytes is necessary. Treatment involves dietician input and supplementation with phosphate.

Notes

- Other physical consequences of anorexia nervosa are:
  - *Gastrointestinal*: Delayed gastric emptying, gastric atrophy, constipation.
  - *Metabolic*: Hypokalaemia, hyponatraemia, hypoglycaemia, hypocalcaemia, hypomagnesaemia, hypercholesterolaemia, deranged thyroid function.
  - *Haematological*: Anaemia, leucopaenia, thrombocytopaenia.
  - *Neurological*: Peripheral neuropathy, cerebral pseudoatrophy, ventricular enlargement.
  - *Physical signs*: Lanugo (thin, fine) body hair, brittle nails, hypothermia.
  - *Musculoskeletal*: Osteoporosis, proximal myopathy.

CHAPTER 3
Organic and substance psychiatry

Dementia I

A. Alzheimer's dementia
B. Creutzfeldt–Jakob disease (CJD)
C. HIV-associated dementia
D. Hypothyroidism
E. Lewy body dementia
F. Neurosyphilis
G. Pick's disease
H. Subdural haematoma
I. Vascular dementia
J. Vitamin B12 deficiency

Select the most appropriate diagnosis from the above that best fits with the following clinical descriptions.

1. A 73-year-old female presents with increasing confusion, lethargy, and disorientation. On examination, she is obese and has a distinctive deep voice. Her pulse is 40 and blood pressure is 110/72. She complains of constipation.

2. An 80-year-old female presents with long-standing dizziness, weakness, and increasing confusion. On examination, she has an ataxic gait with loss of vibration sense and proprioception. Fundoscopic examination reveals optic atrophy.

3. A 50-year-old male is brought to hospital with a severe chest infection. He has word finding difficulties, apathy, and social withdrawal. On examination, he has ataxia, marked tremor, myoclonus, and incoordination. Blood tests reveal decreased lymphocytes.

4. A 60-year-old male presents with grandiose delusions and hypomania, associated with increasing memory problems. On examination, he has brisk reflexes, extensor plantar reflexes, and small pupils that are unreactive to light.

5. A 55-year-old male is brought to hospital by his family. They have noticed that over the last 2 years, the patient's personality has changed and he no longer seems to care about anything. He is disinhibited and easily gets into arguments with others. He constantly repeats the same things and his memory is poor.

Dementia II

A. Alcoholic dementia
B. Alzheimer's dementia
C. HIV-associated dementia
D. Huntington's disease
E. Lewy body dementia
F. Normal pressure hydrocephalus
G. Pick's disease
H. Pseudodementia
I. Vascular dementia
J. Wilson's disease

Select the most appropriate diagnosis from the above that best fits with the following clinical descriptions.

1. A 72-year-old male has been experiencing attacks of confusion, memory problems, and visual hallucinations over the last year. Each episode lasts for a few weeks and he is fine between these episodes; however, with subsequent episodes, his condition seems to be getting worse. His medical history shows blood pressure of 150/101 and he has had transient ischaemic attacks in the past. On examination there is an upgoing plantar.

2. A 78-year-old female presents with episodes of wandering at night. She is unable to look after herself and is no longer able to recognise her family. Her mini-mental state examination score was 19 out of 30.

3. A 60-year-old male is referred to a specialist with cognitive problems. On his arrival it is noted that he has an unsteady gait and his wife also reveals that he has been incontinent.

4. An 82-year-old female is convinced that she sees children playing inside her house. Her daughter noticed that her memory tends to fluctuate and that she has recently developed a mild tremor of her right hand. Physical examination reveals cogwheel rigidity and a shuffling gait. When the doctor looking after her administers a small dose of haloperidol she is found to be very sensitive to this.

5. A 40-year-old male is referred to a specialist because of difficulties with his memory. He admits to feeling increasingly depressed over the last 6 months. There is evidence of psychomotor retardation, and the psychiatric assessment is difficult to carry out as he answers most questions with 'I don't know'.

Medical causes of psychiatric illnesses

A. Acute intermittent porphyria
B. Huntington's chorea
C. Multiple sclerosis
D. Neurosyphilis
E. Pellagra
F. Sporadic CJD
G. Thiamine deficiency
H. Variant CJD
I. Vitamin B12 deficiency
J. Wilson's disease

Select the most appropriate medical condition from the above that best fits with the following clinical descriptions.

1. A 44-year-old African female refugee from a famine stricken area presents with loose stools, cognitive impairment, and itchy, flaky skin. Her diet in Africa consisted of only maize as this was the only available crop. Her mood is also noticeably low with marked apathy. Her family is worried about her, as she seems to have lost her interests and is no longer able to work.

2. A 35-year-old male presents with jaundice and ascites. He has been complaining of tremor of his arms and legs, and has become increasingly irritable. His speech is slurred and he has an ataxic gait. His blood tests show elevated liver enzymes and decreased caeruloplasmin levels.

3. A 35-year-old female presents with painful loss of vision in one eye, weakness of her right arm and leg, uncontrollable spasms of her muscles, constipation, and urinary retention. Her symptoms worsen after she takes a hot bath. Her family have noticed that her memory has deteriorated and she admits to feeling depressed.

4. A 30-year-old female presents with colicky abdominal pain, peripheral neuropathy, bulbar palsies, and psychosis after being prescribed the oral contraceptive pill. Her urine is noted to be deep red after a period of standing.

5. A 25-year-old male is referred to a psychiatrist for anxiety and depressive symptoms. He performs poorly on the mini-mental state examination, and on physical examination he has an ataxic gait with evidence of myoclonus. A CT scan of his head reveals atrophy of the cortex and cerebellum, and he has an abnormal EEG.

Endocrine causes of psychiatric illnesses

A. Addison's disease
B. Cushing's syndrome
C. Diabetes insipidus
D. Diabetes mellitus
E. Hyperparathyroidism
F. Hyperprolactinaemia
G. Hyperthyroidism
H. Hypopituitarism
I. Hypothyroidism
J. Phaeochromocytoma

Select the most appropriate medical condition from the above that best fits with the following clinical descriptions.

1. A 32-year-old male presents to hospital with a severely depressed mood. On examination, he has central obesity with purple stretch marks on his abdomen. He informs that he has recently gained 15 kg in weight and that he tends to bruise easily. His past medical history is significant of a rib fracture he sustained a month ago.

2. A 55-year-old female presents to hospital complaining of feeling depressed and lethargic. She feels that her concentration is decreased and has trouble sleeping at night. On physical examination, she has a left-sided colicky abdominal pain radiating to her groin. She scores 20/30 on mini-mental state examination, losing points for concentration and memory. Her past medical history is significant for a fracture of her humerus.

3. A 25-year-old female presents to her doctor after losing 11 kg in weight. She finds tolerating warm weather difficult, and complains of loose stools and irregular periods. She also feels embarrassed about her hands shaking. Her partner believes that she has become extremely irritable and agitated lately.

4. A 69-year-old female is admitted to hospital because of her low mood. Although she is not losing weight, she feels tired all the time and lacks motivation. Her family are worried about her as she has become increasingly forgetful and has trouble looking after herself. Her physical examination is remarkable for slow reflexes, bradycardia, constipation, and a slow, hoarse voice.

5. A 42-year-old male complains of 'panic attacks' which have become worse recently. He describes that these episodes of anxiety are associated with palpitation, recurrent headaches, and sweating. On examination, he was hypertensive and tachycardic, and his urine revealed raised catecholamine levels.

Alcohol misuse I

A. Acute alcohol withdrawal
B. Alcohol intoxication
C. Alcoholic dementia
D. Alcoholic hallucinosis
E. Delirium tremens
F. Intracranial bleed
G. Korsakoff's psychosis
H. Pathological intoxication
I. Peripheral neuropathy
J. Wernicke's encephalopathy

A 60-year-old male is brought to hospital with fluctuating consciousness and injury to his forehead. He has a history of alcohol abuse. Select the most appropriate item from the above for each of the following presentations.

1. He is emotionally labile, disinhibited, and has an ataxic gait.

2. He is noted to have lateral gaze palsy, nystagmus, and staggering gait. He is confused and disoriented. On admission to the ward, he is treated with high-dose parenteral thiamine, and his condition quickly improves.

3. He denies the existence of the other half of his body.

4. His cognition reveals marked short-term memory loss, confabulation, and labile personality. On review by the psychiatrists, they feel that this condition is hard to reverse.

5. He is noted to have minor tremors in his hands. On testing his cognition, he scores 13/30 on the mini-mental state examination, losing marks on orientation, memory, and registration. His wife confirms that his behaviour has been erratic for the last year, and on some occasion, has wandered off on the street. A CT scan of the brain shows enlarged ventricular space.

Alcohol misuse II

A. Alcohol-induced schizophrenia
B. Alcohol intoxication
C. Alcoholic dementia
D. Alcoholic hallucinosis
E. Cerebellar degeneration
F. Delirium tremens
G. Foetal alcohol syndrome
H. Korsakoff's syndrome
I. Othello syndrome
J. Wernicke's encephalopathy

The following scenarios refer to patients with a history of chronic alcohol abuse. Select the most appropriate item from the above that best describes the clinical descriptions.

1. A 36-year-old female with a long history of alcohol abuse decides to stop drinking without any help. She appeared to be coping well but on the 4th day of total abstinence, she becomes increasingly agitated and starts screaming that small animals are flying around her. She is sweating profusely and appears disoriented.

2. A 56-year-old male with a long history of alcohol abuse complains that over the last year, he has been hearing strange noises in his apartment despite living alone. These seem to happen even when he is not drinking and initially started as buzzing noises, but in the last 2 months, have become clear voices. He claims that his dead father is telling him that he is a failure.

3. A 23-year-old male with a history of alcohol and drug abuse was referred to the forensic team because of his offences relating to damage to property and arrests for theft. His history indicates that he had delayed motor development and was diagnosed with a mild learning disability. His impulse control had been poor and he was expelled from school at age 15 years. He has never been able to keep a stable employment.

4. A 45-year-old male with a long history of alcohol abuse was recently arrested for attacking his neighbour. According to him, he had ongoing suspicions that his wife was having an affair

with the neighbour and meticulously confronted her every night. He knew that his suspicions were correct when he spotted his wife saying hello to the neighbour.

5. A 43-year-old female with a long history of alcohol abuse completes alcohol detoxification but still presents with an ataxic gait and scanning speech. Her movements appear to be uncoordinated but there is no evidence of confusion or ophthalmoplegia. On further physical examination, areas of decreased sensation were noted on her legs.

Substance misuse I

A. Benzodiazepine withdrawal
B. Cannabis intoxication
C. Cannabis withdrawal
D. Cocaine intoxication
E. Cocaine withdrawal
F. Lysergic acid diethylamide (LSD) intoxication
G. Methylenedioxymethamphetamine (MDMA) intoxication
H. Opiate intoxication
I. Opiate withdrawal
J. Psilocybin withdrawal

Select the most appropriate item from the above that best fits with the following clinical descriptions.

1. A 23-year-old female is brought into hospital after having a seizure. She is hypertensive, tachycardic, and noted to have a nosebleed and dilated pupils. She claims to be a movie star and that everyone is preventing her from marrying someone famous. Her friend however explains that she works as a sex worker in order to finance her drug habit.

2. An 18-year-old male gives a 2-month history of becoming more withdrawn, acting inappropriately, and showing cognitive difficulties. According to his mother, there is a history of episodic panic attacks and anxiety, with occasional paranoia. On examination, he is noted to have a cough and blood shot eyes.

3. A 36-year-old male with a history of polysubstance abuse is found to be sweating profusely, agitated, and tachycardic. He claims to 'see the colour red' while listening to an orchestral performance. On questioning, he recalls having vivid flashbacks and nightmares from time to time over the last few months.

4. A 32-year-old male is brought to hospital complaining of abdominal cramps, diarrhoea, vomiting, and headaches. On physical examination, he is found to be extremely irritable, agitated, sweaty, and shaking. There is also evidence of a large abscess on his groin and large dilated pupils.

5. A 40-year-old female presents to hospital complaining of feeling 'on the edge', and that her head feels 'like a balloon'. She says that the world is spinning around her, and is unable to walk normally as she feels like she is walking on cotton wool. She also complains of high-pitched noise in her ear and hypersensitivity to light and sound.

Substance misuse II

A. Alcohol
B. Amyl nitrites
C. Cannabis
D. Cocaine
E. Gamma-hydroxy-butyrate (GHB)
F. Heroin
G. Ketamine
H. Khat
I. Phencyclidine (PCP)
J. Psilocybin

Select the most appropriate item from the above for each of the following statements.

1. This drug is taken through inhalation and produces mild euphoria, slurred speech, tachycardia, vasodilation, and occasional perceptual distortion within seconds. It also causes relaxation of the smooth muscles, with some reporting heightened sexual awareness. It is not classified by the UK Misuse of Drugs Act.

2. This drug is a mild stimulant available as plant leaves and usually chewed in order to produce a sense of excitement and euphoria. Its use is socially accepted in the Somali community and the drug is legally available in the UK. Occasionally heavy use may mimic a psychotic episode.

3. This is usually taken in liquid form, and takes roughly 15–30 minutes for it to have an effect. It produces a sense of intoxication, euphoria, and sexual disinhibition. Side effects include nausea, vomiting, seizures, and death from respiratory depression. It is emerging as a 'date rape drug' and designated Class C in the UK.

4. This drug comes as a white powder that can be sniffed to cause a sense of dissociation, but in larger amounts causes hallucination and sensory distortion. It is also available in liquid form which may be ingested or injected intramuscularly. Rarely, it can also cause flashbacks, psychotic episodes, and amnesic syndromes. It is designated Class C as of 2006 in the UK.

5. This drug is taken orally and produces a sense of heightened sensations, perceptual abnormalities, and euphoria. Cognitive effects include distorted thinking and occasional paranoia. It may produce dizziness, diarrhoea, abdominal cramps, tachycardia, pupil dilation, and lacrimation. They are not usually associated with dependence or withdrawal, and tolerance develops quickly. Effects usually last for 4–6 hours. It is designated as Class A in the UK when prepared for use.

Epilepsy

A. Absence seizure
B. Atonic seizure
C. Complex partial seizure
D. Febrile seizure
E. Myoclonic seizure
F. Pseudoseizure
G. Secondary generalised seizure
H. Simple partial seizure
I. Tonic-clonic seizure
J. Unclassified seizure

The following patients present with altered behaviours associated with a seizure. Select the most appropriate item from the above for each of the following statements.

1. A 23-year-old male starts shouting incomprehensible words and looks apprehensive. He appears to be hyperventilating, then falls on the floor. His muscles stiffen, and then he starts jerking and twitching his arms and legs. On regaining consciousness, he is found to have bitten his tongue and emptied his bladder. He appears perplexed.

2. A 26-year-old female with a past psychiatric history of border-line personality disorder is admitted to the psychiatric unit following an overdose. While on the ward, she collapses on the floor and starts jerking her body bilaterally. On regaining consciousness, she apologises to the nurse for her seizure.

3. A 20-year-old female complains that she can smell onions, then stares blankly into space. She subsequently loses consciousness but quickly recovers after 4 minutes. She appears perplexed for several minutes after the incident. She has no recollection of the event.

4. A 19-year-old male is working at the check out counter at the local supermarket, but while on duty, he stares blankly into space and does not respond to his customers. After 10 seconds, he continues with his duty with no problems. Apparently, he has had regular lapses in his concentration since he was a small child.

5. A 12-year-old male was eating dinner with his family. While trying to drink a cup of tea, he suddenly throws the cup backwards without any warning. He could not explain what had happened or why he did it. His past medical history is negative, including that for Tourette's syndrome.

Answers

Dementia I

1. **D.** Hypothyroidism is a reversible cause of dementia and should be excluded in everyone presenting with cognitive impairment in those over the age of 65 years. Clinical signs and symptoms are hypotension, bradycardia, cold intolerance, confusion, and constipation.

2. **J.** Vitamin B12 deficiency can cause subacute combined degeneration of the spinal cord, which is characterised by peripheral neuropathy and loss of joint position and vibration sense. It can also cause dementia. Causes include pernicious anaemia, gastrectomy, Crohn's disease, and dietary deficiency.

3. **C.** HIV-associated dementia is an AIDS-defining illness and its clinical features include dementia (subcortical), motor abnormalities (such as tremor, ataxia, and myoclonus), and mood disturbance (such as depression, agitation, and mania). CT or MRI scans show atrophy. Other HIV-associated illnesses such as pneumocystic carinii pneumonia may also be present at time of presentation.

4. **F.** Neurosyphilis can present with *meningovascular syphilis* (cranial nerve palsies, focal deficits from gumma expansion, raised intracranial pressure, delirium, and dementia) after 1–5 years, *'general paralysis of the insane'* (euphoria, mania, grandiosity, psychotic symptoms, personality changes, and dementia) after 5–25 years, or *tabes dorsalis* (demyelination of the dorsal roots leading to lightening pains, loss of proprioception, paraesthesia, and Charcot's joints) after 8–12 years. A characteristic sign seen in neurosyphilis is the Argyll Robertson pupils, which are small bilateral pupils which constrict on accommodation but not to light.

5. **G.** Pick's disease is associated with frontal lobe syndrome (personality changes, social disinhibition), and speech and language abnormalities such as echolalia and perseveration. Cognitive impairment occurs later. There is atrophy of the frontal and temporal lobes. Pick bodies (irregular neurofilament inclusions) and balloon cells are seen histopathologically.

Notes

- A subdural haematoma may present with changes in consciousness, headache, and dementia, often weeks or months after the injury causing the bleed.
- Dementias are often referred to as cortical or subcortical.
  - Subcortical dementias (e.g. Huntington's disease, progressive supranuclear palsy, HIV-associated dementia) usually affect the basal ganglia and are associated with a slowing of thought processes (bradyphrenia), abnormal movements, and changes in personality. Dysarthria, incoordination, and psychomotor retardation may be present.
  - Cortical dementias (e.g. Alzheimer's dementia, Pick's disease) are more likely to present with problems with memory, visuospatial problems, agnosia, apraxia, aphasia, and frontal lobe abnormalities. Mood is more likely to be euthymic, with an absence of dysarthria and abnormal movements. Coordination is usually normal.

Dementia II

1. I. Vascular dementia is the second most common dementia and accounts for 20% of cases. Features include a sudden onset of symptoms, a stepwise deterioration with periods of intervening stability, and cardiovascular risk factors. Deficits are unevenly distributed with some functions being affected while others are spared. Insight and personality are usually preserved until later on. Depression, a labile affect, and confusion are common. Physical signs include unilateral spastic weakness of limbs, increased tendon reflexes, an extended plantar response, and pseudobulbar palsy.

2. B. Alzheimer's dementia is the most common cause of dementia accounting for 70% of cases. Symptoms develop gradually and early symptoms include poor short-term memory, wandering, irritability, and deterioration in self-care. Receptive and expressive aphasia, apraxia, and agnosia may occur. Depression, psychotic symptoms, behavioural disturbances, and personality change may occur. CT scan of the brain may show cortical atrophy, which is marked over the parietal and temporal lobes with ventricular dilatation.

3. F. Normal pressure hydrocephalus presents with a triad of cognitive impairment, ataxia, and urinary incontinence. Lumbar puncture reveals normal CSF pressure, and CT scan of the brain reveals the presence of dilated ventricles. Half of the cases are due to mechanical obstruction to the flow of CSF across the meninges. Treatment is with a ventriculo-peritoneal shunt.

4. E. Lewy body dementia accounts for 15–20% of cases and is characterised by dementia, parkinsonian features, visual hallucinations (often of people or animals), fluctuating cognitive function, and episodes of confusion. There is a marked sensitivity to antipsychotics. Patients may present with recurrent falls due to unsteadiness of gait.

5. H. Some patients with depression may present with cognitive difficulties resulting in a lower than expected score on the minimental state examination, and this is known as pseudodementia. Pseudodementia is difficult to differentiate from dementia, and it should be suspected if there are biological symptoms of depression and deficits such as apraxia or agnosia are absent. Concentration is particularly affected. Individuals often respond to answers on the mini-mental state examination with 'I don't know'. Such difficulties usually resolve following antidepressant treatment.

Notes
- Dementia occurs in 20–30% of patients with Parkinson's disease (PD). It may be difficult to differentiate PD from Lewy body dementia, but generally if the motor symptoms precede the onset of dementia by 12 months a diagnosis of PD is given. Lewy bodies are present in both disorders.

Medical causes of psychiatric illnesses
1. E. Pellagra is a rare condition caused by nicotinic acid deficiency and is characterised by the classic triad of diarrhoea, dementia, and dermatitis, although not all symptoms are usually present together. Other features include neuropathy, depression, ataxia, and seizures. Nicotinic acid deficiency is seen in those with poor diet consisting solely of maize, usually among rural South Americans, those from famine stricken areas, prisoners, and sometimes in chronic alcoholics.

2. J. Wilson's disease results in the accumulation of copper in the brain and the liver. Urinary copper is increased and serum caeruloplasmin is decreased. Features include tremor, dyskinesia, dysarthria, ataxia, and Kayser–Fleischer rings on the cornea. Psychiatric features include mood disturbances, dementia, and rarely psychosis.

3. C. Multiple sclerosis is characterised by plaques of demyelination throughout the CNS. It may present with motor and sensory symptoms, bladder and bowel symptoms, sexual dysfunction, cerebellar signs and symptoms, visual problems, depression, dementia, and psychosis. Symptoms may worsen due to increased temperature, and this is known as Uhthoff's sign. Lhermitte's sign may also be present (paraesthesia in the limbs on flexing the neck).

4. A. Acute intermittent porphyria is an autosomal dominant condition and attacks may be precipitated by many drugs including anaesthetic drugs, certain antibiotics, oral hypoglycaemic drugs, and the oral contraceptive pill. It is characterised by raised urinary porphobilinogens (red urine). Other psychiatric symptoms include depression and delirium.

5. H. CJD is a rare prion disease characterised by parietal lobe symptoms, cortical blindness, myoclonic jerks, speech disturbance, and epileptic fits. The variant CJD type mainly affects young males in their 20s, and sensory symptoms (pain, numbness, and burning sensation) and psychiatric symptoms (anxiety and depressive symptoms) are usually the reasons for presenting to a doctor. The course of illness is 1–2 years, and patients usually develop personality changes and dementia.

Notes
• Sporadic CJD has an age of onset of 50–70 years with equal sex distribution. There are cerebellar and extrapyramidal signs, myoclonus, and a rapidly progressing dementia. Prions are seen primarily in the cortex, and the EEG is characterised by periodic triphasic complexes. Positive family history is seen in 15%. Death occurs within a year.

- Huntington's disease is a rare autosomal disorder caused by a gene defect that results in the expansion of the trinucleotide sequence CAG. It presents with chorea, personality changes, psychosis, and progressive dementia.

- Neurosyphilis may present with the 'general paralysis of the insane', in which the patient displays grandiose delusions, mania, dementia, and personality change. A significant finding on neurological examination would be the Argyll Robertson pupil, which accommodates but is slow to react to light ('prostitute pupil').

Endocrine causes of psychiatric conditions

1. **B.** The diagnosis here is Cushing's syndrome, which results from excess production of cortisol. Causes of Cushing's syndrome include a pituitary tumour (Cushing's disease), adrenal adenoma or carcinoma, and iatrogenic (treatment with steroids). Symptoms include weight gain, amenorrhoea and other menstrual abnormalities, muscle weakness, impotence in men, hirsutism in women, fractures, depression, euphoria, and psychotic symptoms. Signs include purple abdominal striae, bruising, myopathy, osteoporosis, hypertension, and hyperglycaemia.

2. **E.** Hyperparathyroidism manifests with increased serum calcium due to the increased levels of parathyroid hormone. Signs and symptoms are thus secondary to raised calcium, and are commonly known as 'stones (kidney), groans (abdominal pain and myalgia), and moans (psychiatric)'. Psychiatric symptoms include depression, delirium, and cognitive impairment.

3. **G.** Causes of hyperthyroidism include Graves' disease, toxic adenoma, multinodular goitre, and subacute thyroiditis. Symptoms include weight loss, heat intolerance, sweating, tremor, irritability, anxiety, and rarely delirium and psychosis. Signs include tremor, tachycardia, atrial fibrillation, palmar erythema, and lid lag. In Graves' disease, exophthalmos, thyroid bruit, and thyroid acropachy may occur.

4. **I.** Hypothyroidism may occur due to underactivity of the thyroid, or less commonly, due to disease of the hypothalamus or pituitary. The most common cause is autoimmune disease. It can present with a range of symptoms including lethargy, weight gain, cold intolerance, constipation, and menorrhagia. Signs

include dry skin, loss of eyebrows, and slow relaxing reflexes. It may present with psychiatric symptoms such as depression, dementia, or psychosis.

5. **J.** Phaeochromocytoma is a rare tumour that produces catecholamines. The majority of tumours are in the adrenal medulla. Characteristic features include episodes of hypertension, palpitations, chest tightness, restlessness, anxiety, sweating, headache, pallor, and weakness. It can be detected by measuring urine catecholamine levels.

Notes

• Addison's disease is a rare condition caused by destruction of the adrenal cortex, leading to reduced cortisol, aldosterone, and androgen production. The majority of cases (80%) are caused by autoantibodies against the adrenal cortex. It has an insidious onset and may present with lethargy, depression, anorexia, weight loss, hypotension, and hyperpigmentation.

• Hyperprolactinaemia can result from iatrogenic causes (antipsychotics), prolactinoma, polycystic ovary syndrome, chronic renal failure, and hypothyroidism. It manifests with menstrual disruption, galactorrhoea, loss of libido, and impotence.

• Causes of hypopituitarism include hypophysectomy, pituitary adenoma, and irradiation. Signs and symptoms occur due to deficiency of anterior pituitary hormones (e.g. FSH, LH, TSH). Psychiatric symptoms include depression, cognitive impairment, and rarely delirium.

Alcohol misuse I

1. **B.** Features of alcohol intoxication include elevated mood, disinhibition, impaired judgement, unsteady gait, slurred speech, labile mood, aggression, nystagmus, and ataxia.

2. **J.** The four characteristics of Wernicke's encephalopathy are confusion, ophthalmoplegia (usually VIth nerve palsy resulting in lateral gaze), nystagmus, and ataxia. Peripheral neuropathy may also be present. Treatment is with parenteral thiamine given in the form of intramuscular Pabrinex, two ampoules twice a day for 3–7 days. If left untreated, over 80% of cases go on to develop Korsakoff's psychosis.

3. F. Intracranial bleed can present with neurological deficits, and in this scenario, the patient is presenting with sensory inattention. This is due to a lesion on the contralateral parietal lobe.

4. G. Korsakoff's psychosis is characterised by an inability to form new memories. There is relative preservation of other intellectual functioning (such as working memory) and patients may confabulate (fabrication of recollection of experiences in clear consciousness in order to fill in gaps in memory). This is thought to be an irreversible condition.

5. C. Alcoholic dementia is characterised by mild to moderate cognitive difficulties such as impaired memory and judgment with personal and social neglect. It is associated with ventricular enlargement and atrophy in the frontal lobes. In a small number of cases, symptoms may improve on abstinence.

Notes
- In the UK, measure of alcohol is made in *units*, where one unit is equivalent to roughly 10 mL of pure ethanol. This is equivalent to a small glass of wine, or half a pint of beer. In the UK, the maximum number of recommended units of alcohol per week is 21 units for men and 14 units for women.

- Pathological intoxication (*mania a potu*) refers to an alcohol intoxication state characterised by violent and disinhibited behaviour that occurs after drinking only small quantities of alcohol.

- Alcohol withdrawal in its initial stages presents with coarse tremor, sweating, insomnia, tachycardia, agitation, and nausea. There is a strong compulsion to drink and occurs roughly 4–12 hours after the last drink.
  - Roughly 10% of alcoholic withdrawals are complicated by grand mal seizures, which may occur 6–48 hours after the last drink.

Alcohol misuse II
1. F. Delirium tremens is a medical emergency and should be treated promptly. It occurs most commonly in patients with severe dependency and evidence of liver damage is seen in up to

90% of cases. Hallucinations are characteristically of little people or animals ('Lilliputian' hallucinations). This condition may be associated with dehydration, electrolyte abnormalities, and infection, which should be treated. Mortality rate is 5–10%.

2. D. Alcoholic hallucinosis is associated with chronic alcohol abuse and characterised by hallucinations (usually auditory) occurring in clear consciousness and when sober. Auditory hallucinations may be elementary in nature initially, but may progress to become clear, second-person voices, which are usually derogatory in nature. Most cases improve following abstinence and rarely persist for more than 6 months. Differential diagnosis includes delirium tremens and schizophrenia.

3. G. Foetal alcohol syndrome is one of the major causes of learning disability and it is estimated that 10–20% of mild learning disability may be due to maternal drinking. Physical features include epicanthic folds, maxillary hypoplasia, short stature, cleft palate, poor visual acuity, and hearing problems. Affected individuals go on to develop social difficulties (such as unemployment) and substance abuse due to poor impulse control.

4. I. Othello syndrome consists of a delusion of jealousy that one's partner has been or is unfaithful. It is a recognised complication of chronic alcohol use but also seen in other psychotic illnesses. The individual goes to great lengths to obtain evidence for the affair, and the nature of the evidence in which the delusion is based makes it a delusion. It can be associated with violence to the partner or the alleged individual in the affair.

5. E. Cerebellar degeneration may occur with chronic alcohol misuse and may present with incoordination, ataxia, and scanning speech. The patient in this vignette is clearly showing signs of this, as well as peripheral neuropathy (decreased sensation) in the legs.

Notes

• Psychotic disorders may be induced by chronic alcohol use and manifest with delusions of persecution, but a diagnosis of 'alcohol-induced schizophrenia' *per se* does not exist.

Substance misuse I

1. **D.** Cocaine is a stimulant ('upper') and may be snorted, or dissolved and injected. 'Crack' or free-base cocaine may be smoked. Effects include increased energy, euphoria, increased confidence, and decreased need for sleep. Crack cocaine is associated with intense 'highs' followed by rapid 'lows'. Harmful effects include arrhythmias, hypertension, necrosis of the nasal septum, and psychotic symptoms.
   • Withdrawal effects of cocaine manifests as the opposite of intoxication, and symptoms include the 'crash', fatigue, lack of pleasure, anxiety, irritability, and sleeplessness.

2. **B.** Cannabis may be smoked or taken orally when mixed with food. Effects include a mild euphoria, relaxation, altered sense of time, and increased appetite. Regular use can cause psychotic symptoms, anxiety, depressive symptoms, and lack of motivation.
   • Cannabis withdrawal is seen in heavy users who stop use abruptly. Symptoms include sleep disturbance, irritability, loss of appetite, and diarrhoea. This usually settles within a week.

3. **F.** LSD is a hallucinogen which may affect the body for 8–12 hours, and the effects include euphoria, visual distortions, and synaesthesia (stimulus in one sensory modality is perceived by another sensory modality such as seeing or tasting music). Physical effects such as hyperthermia, tachycardia, pupil dilation, and smooth muscle contraction are also seen. Secondary psycho-emotional effects, including feelings of dissociation, flashbacks, and mood disturbance, may occur up to 72 hours after ingestion, or sometimes more. It is taken orally, usually through paper blotted with the solution.

4. **I.** Opiate withdrawal is associated with craving, agitation, dilated pupils, yawning, diarrhoea, nausea and vomiting, abdominal cramps, and goose pimples.
   • Opiate is commonly available as heroin, which can be injected, ingested, or smoked ('chasing the dragon'). It acts on the opioid receptors in the brain and produces a sense of euphoria. Signs and symptoms of use include miosis (pupillary constriction), analgesia, hypotension, bradycardia, and respiratory depression.

5. A. Benzodiazepines are anxiolytic agents which include lorazepam and diazepam. Withdrawal symptoms include tinnitus, rebound insomnia, tremor, dizziness, restlessness, depersonalisation, sensory disturbances, and rarely psychotic symptoms and seizures.

Notes

- MDMA is commonly known as ecstasy or 'pill' and remains popular in the clubbing and rave scene. It produces a sense of euphoria, openness, love, and heightened self-awareness. Physical signs include nystagmus, dilated pupils, loss of appetite, teeth-grinding, and dehydration. It is a stimulant which can raise the body's core temperature and may lead to fatal hyperpyrexia. Over-ingestion of liquid to counteract potential dehydration can also cause water intoxication and hyponatraemia, which in itself may be fatal.

Substance misuse II

1. B. Amyl nitrites are found in a variety of products including glue, solvents, lighter fluid, extinguishers, aerosols, paint, and petrol. They are rapidly absorbed through inhalation or sniffing. Acute harmful effects include arrhythmias, aspiration, and local irritation. Other chronic effects include kidney and liver damage. It is known by the street name of poppers.

2. H. The active ingredient in khat is a chemical known as cathinone, which has amphetamine-like properties. It is grown in large amounts in some African countries, particularly Somalia. Consumption leads to mild euphoria, excitement, and hyperactivity. Chronic heavy use can also trigger mania and mimic a psychotic episode. Although its use is restricted in large parts of Europe and North America, there are no UK regulations restricting its use or sale.

3. E. GHB is a CNS depressant that can be used as an anaesthetic and hypnotic. Its street name includes liquid ecstasy, juice, and fantasy. In small doses, it produces a sense of euphoria, increased sexuality, and increased confidence. However, in higher doses, it depresses the body system by inducing nausea, drowsiness, visual disturbances, and decreased respiration. This may lead to unconsciousness and eventual death. Withdrawal symptoms have been reported and include hallucination, insomnia, agitation, dysphoria, muscle aches, and tremors.

4. G. Ketamine is used as an anaesthetic in humans and animals. Its hallucinatory experiences are typically short lasting and usually occur in the absence of sensory stimulation. Its longer-term effects include dizziness, incoordination, and a sense of detachment. Due to its 'mellow' effect, users can quickly become dependent.

5. J. Psilocybin (psychedelic mushrooms) produces sensory disturbances similar to that of LSD in that users experience hallucination (visual and auditory), enhanced perceptions, euphoric bliss, and relaxation, but the duration of effect is shorter (LSD lasting up to 72 hours, while psilocybin lasting around 6 hours). Users often maintain awkward postures as they are unable to feel fatigue or perceive the sense of time.

Notes
- PCP is a hallucinogen commonly seen in the USA and known by names such as 'angel dust'. Physical signs include nystagmus, loss of balance, raised body temperature, and fluctuation of blood pressure. Withdrawal symptoms occur in chronic use and include craving and depression. People who are experiencing 'trips' on PCP may engage in reckless activities such as running into cars, jumping out of windows, and punching down walls as they supposedly do not feel pain.

Epilepsy
1. I. Atonic-clonic seizure is also known as a grand mal seizure. It is characterised by a sudden onset, loss of consciousness, and stiffening of limbs followed by jerking of limbs. It is associated with urinary incontinence and tongue biting. Confusion is usually seen afterwards.

2. F. Pseudoseizures may occur as part of a dissociative disorder. Features include a high frequency of attacks (usually in the presence of others), an atypical pattern to the seizure (such as a gradual onset, rigidity with random struggling, talking, or screaming during the attack), and individuals rarely pass urine or bite their tongue. They are often precipitated by emotional disturbance. The EEG is normal during the attack and prolactin is not raised after the attack (normally raised after a true seizure).

3. C. Complex partial seizures have a focal onset, which usually manifest as an aura, and progress to loss of consciousness. They may also have automatic movements during the seizures in which the individual loses touch with the surrounding. Post-ictal confusion is common.

4. **A.** An absence seizure is also known as a petit mal seizure. Characteristically the individual stops talking mid-sentence for a few seconds but then continues from where he or she has left off. The EEG shows characteristic 'three per second spikes'.

5. **E.** Myoclonic seizures are characterised by the presence of brief, involuntary twitching of a muscle or group of muscles. Patients with this condition may be thrown suddenly to the floor or there may be a violent jerk of one of the limbs.

Notes

- Epilepsy is a common neurological condition characterised by the presence of unprovoked epileptic seizures or fits. These seizures can be broadly classified as:
  - Generalised (originating from both hemisphere) or partial (one hemisphere).
  - Complex (loss of consciousness) or simple (no loss of consciousness).

- Simple partial seizures can present in a number of ways depending on the origin of the seizure, but consciousness is always retained. Common presentations of temporal lobe epilepsy are altered perceptions (e.g. hallucinations, déjà vu), autonomic effects (e.g. vertigo, dizziness), cognitive abnormalities (e.g. speech disturbances), and affective changes (e.g. anxiety).

- Partial seizures may occasionally spread to both hemispheres, and can lead to secondary generalised seizures.

- Atonic seizures are associated with loss of tone and are also known as 'drop attacks'.

- Febrile seizures present with generalised convulsions resulting from raised body temperature, and occur during a fever in young children. They may predispose to future epilepsy.

- Psychiatric symptoms occur more commonly in epilepsy compared to the general population, including an increased risk of anxiety disorders, depression, suicide, and psychotic disorders.

CHAPTER 4

Developmental disorders and other clinical syndromes

Psychiatric disorders in children I

A. Asperger's syndrome
B. Autism
C. Conduct disorder
D. Generalised anxiety disorder
E. Hyperkinetic disorder
F. Manic episode
G. Obsessive-compulsive disorder (OCD)
H. Oppositional defiant disorder
I. Separation anxiety disorder
J. Tourette's syndrome

Select the most likely diagnosis from the above for each of the following statements.

1. A 7-year-old male is difficult to manage at home and at school. His teacher reports that he frequently runs around the classroom and cannot remain in his seat for more than a few minutes. He has had a number of accidents in the classroom and on the playground, resulting in cuts and bruises on his body. He cannot focus his attention on one task and is easily distracted. The other children are annoyed by his inability to wait his turn when playing games and his intrusion during conversations.

2. A 5-year-old male has recently started school but has not been able to keep up in class due to his limited range of vocabulary. The teacher is concerned about his lack of interest in other children and his tendency to play on his own. He shows little eye

contact when others address him and does not initiate conversation with others. His mother reports that he has a strict bedtime ritual, which he performs every night and becomes angry if it is disrupted. He also has tantrums if the layout of his bedroom is altered in any way.

3. A 6-year-old male complains of feeling sick with stomach ache during school days and refuses to go to school. He cries if his mother attempts to leave him under any circumstance. He finds it difficult to go to bed without his mother being by his side and frequently gets up at night to check on her. When questioned about this, he says that he is worried that something terrible will happen to her and that he will never see her again. These symptoms have developed since his parents divorced 6 months ago.

4. An 11-year-old female spends 3 hours in the evening checking that the locks, taps, and light switches have been switched off and rearranges the furniture in her room. She must perform a strict washing ritual as she fears that her parents will come to harm otherwise.

5. A 7-year-old male is frequently rude and argumentative towards his teachers. He becomes easily annoyed by others and is disruptive and disobeys classroom rules. However, he has not been aggressive towards other children and does have a few friends. He appears to have no problems at home.

Psychiatric disorders in children II

A. Antisocial personality disorder
B. Attachment disorder
C. Chronic tic disorder
D. Conduct disorder
E. Elective mutism
F. Encopresis
G. Enuresis
H. Gilles de la Tourette's syndrome
I. Hyperkinetic disorder
J. Oppositional defiant disorder

Select the most likely diagnosis from the above for each of the following statements.

1. A 9-year-old male presents with motor tics of jumping and hitting himself and vocal tics of barking, throat clearing, and shouting of obscenities. These symptoms are exacerbated at times of stress and have been present for over 3 years.

2. A 9-year-old male regularly wets his bed several nights per week, which began shortly after the separation of his parents. Since the separation, his mother noticed that he has been more irritable than usual.

3. A 5-year-old female has not had any problems with development. On starting school, however, the teacher notices that she has not been participating in class and does not talk to her peers. However, she speaks normally to her siblings and parents at home.

4. A 7-year-old male has been repeatedly soiling his underwear since his grandfather's death. He does not soil himself at night, but appears to do so while he is at school and while playing games at home. He has also been depositing his faeces behind the sofa and underneath his bed. His parents were inconsistent in toilet training him.

5. A 12-year-old male regularly gets into trouble at school for bullying and physical aggression towards other children. He

frequently truants from school and has been issued with an Antisocial Behavioural Order for setting fire to some vehicles in his neighbourhood. He also has a history of stealing from shops, cruelty to animals, and has mugged several elderly women.

Genetic disorders associated with learning disability

A. Angelman syndrome
B. Down's syndrome
C. Edward's syndrome
D. Fragile X syndrome
E. Galactosaemia
F. Lesch–Nyhan syndrome
G. Phenylketonuria
H. Prader–Willi syndrome
I. Tay–Sachs disease
J. Tuberous sclerosis

The following patients have all been diagnosed with a learning disability. Select the most appropriate genetic condition from the above for each of the following statements.

1. A sociable 5-year-old female is noted to have a protuding tongue, epicanthic folds of her eyelids, and brushfield spots on the iris. She also has broad hands with a single palmer crease and widely spaced first and second toes. She suffers from a congenital heart defect and hypotonia, and has a moderate learning disability.

2. A morbidly obese 11-year-old male has difficulty controlling his anger and has an insatiable appetite resulting in overeating. He attends a special school as he was diagnosed with mild learning disability when he was younger. On examination, he is short in stature and has small testes.

3. A 7-year-old female has severe epilepsy and moderate learning disability. She is noted to have flesh coloured patches of skin over her lumbosacral area and ash leaf-shaped areas of hypopigmented skin. Several members of her family including her father and one of her siblings are affected.

4. An 8-year-old female with a learning disability has fair hair and blue eyes. She suffers from eczema and epilepsy, and has been eating a special diet since she was a baby. This was recommended by the specialist in order to prevent further deterioration of her condition.

5. A 12-year-old male with a moderate learning disability was brought to hospital because of repeated episodes of an epileptic seizure. On examination, he has a long narrow head with long ears and large testes. He appears shy and avoids eye-to-eye contact. Assessment by a specialist indicated that abnormal CGG trinucleotide expansion is responsible for this condition.

Psychiatric syndromes I

A. Chronic fatigue syndrome
B. Cotard's syndrome
C. Couvade's syndrome
D. De Clerambault's syndrome
E. Delusional misidentification syndrome
F. Ekbom's syndrome
G. Folie a deux
H. Ganser's syndrome
I. Munchausen's syndrome
J. Othello syndrome

Select the most appropriate diagnosis from the above that best fits with the following clinical descriptions.

1. A 38-year-old married journalist, who has a well paid job for a newspaper, often turns to alcohol for stress relief. One day, his wife returns home from work wearing a miniskirt, and he is convinced that she is having an affair and aggressively confronts her.

2. A 30-year-old unemployed male who is a polysubstance abuser presents to the local hospital with multiple self-inflicted cuts on his arms and legs, complaining that there are 'bugs' underneath his skin and that he has been trying to get rid of them with no success.

3. A 28-year-old female goes to a concert as she believes that a member of a rock group is in love with her. She claims that they have been dating together for 2 years, when she first ran into him on the streets and their eyes met. She says that he has not been in contact with her lately as he has been busy with the tour.

4. A 23-year-old male was admitted to hospital 2 days ago complaining of headaches, aching muscles, joint pains, and lethargy. Differential diagnoses included anaemia and viral infections, but both were ruled out. The patient has not made any progress since being admitted, and still complains of unrefreshing sleep and drowsiness. Apparently, he has always been 'weak' since he was a small child.

5. A 70-year-old male was admitted to hospital compulsorily as his family noted that he had become increasingly inactive and withdrawn. On interview, he is not spontaneous, requires a lot of encouragement, and has poor concentration. He has been refusing any oral intake for the last 5 days, as he believes that he is 'dead' and as such, does not require any food.

Psychiatric syndromes II

A. Capgras' syndrome
B. Cotard's syndrome
C. Couvade's syndrome
D. De Clerambault's syndrome
E. Ekbom's syndrome
F. Folie a deux
G. Fregoli's syndrome
H. Ganser's syndrome
I. Othello syndrome
J. Pseudocyesis

Select the most appropriate item from the above for each of the following statements.

1. A 35-year-old male becomes anxious about his wife's pregnancy and develops morning sickness, abdominal pains, and food cravings.

2. A 45-year-old female believes that her husband has been replaced by an impostor who is an exact double of her husband.

3. A 30-year-old male awaiting a court trial in prison complains to the prison nurse that he is hearing voices in his head telling him to die. He is subsequently assessed by a psychiatrist, but his consciousness was found to be fluctuating throughout the interview. On examination of his cognitive abilities, he answered that camels had six legs and the sky is green.

4. A 58-year-old female is looking after her 55-year-old sister who has a learning disability and is very dependant. The older sister has a diagnosis of schizophrenia and believes that her neighbours are constantly spying on them. The younger sister also believes this. When the older sister is admitted to hospital, the delusion in the younger sister rapidly resolves.

5. A 60-year-old female believes that the police officer who asked her a question on the street is in fact her neighbour. Although she has never seen him before, she believes that her neighbour has transformed himself into an officer in order to get her bank account password.

Culture bound syndromes

A. Amok
B. Ataque de nervios
C. Brain fag
D. Dhat
E. Koro
F. Latah
G. Pibliotoq
H. Susto
I. Taijin kyofusho
J. Windigo

Select the most likely diagnosis from the above for each of the following statements.

1. A 42-year-old male of South East Asian origin believes that his penis is retracting into his abdomen and will disappear. He believes that this is an indication of impending death.

2. A 27-year-old male of Native American origin believes that he has undergone a transformation and has become a cannibal.

3. A 35-year-old male of South Asian origin presents with a period of withdrawal followed by indiscriminate homicidal behaviour, during which he kills others and himself.

4. A 50-year-old female of Inuit origin presents with a period of intense excitement, which is followed by apparent seizures and a transient coma.

5. A 37-year-old female of Malaysian origin has a frightening experience and presents with echolalia, echopraxia, and automatic obedience.

Answers

Psychiatric disorders in children I

1. **E.** Hyperkinetic disorder is described by ICD-10 and its DSM-IV equivalent is attention deficit hyperactivity disorder (ADHD). It is characterised by the presence of hyperactivity, impulsivity, and inattention that is developmentally inappropriate, and all three need to be present for an ICD-10 diagnosis. These symptoms need to be present before the age of 7 years. Hyperkinetic disorder has a prevalence of 1% in the UK (3% in the USA due to diagnostic differences). Most children have other comorbid disorders such as conduct disorders, specific learning difficulties, substance misuse, and depression. Assessment should include interviewing the child and parents separately and then together, and collateral information should be obtained from school and other agencies involved. Connor's rating scale can be used to objectively measure symptoms in order to arrive at a diagnosis.

2. **B.** Autism is a pervasive developmental disorder. The age of onset for autism is usually before the age of 3 years. A diagnosis of autism requires an impairment in social interaction (e.g. gaze, social reciprocity, peer relationships), social communication (e.g. delay in language and abnormalities in speech), and a restricted and stereotyped pattern of interests, behaviours, and activities (e.g. rituals, routines).
   - Up to 70% of the individuals may have learning disabilities.
   - Behavioural problems associated with autism include ADHD, OCD, and aggression. A minority of patients may have isolated abilities. Treatment involves behavioural interventions and appropriate educational placement. Medication is rarely used, although risperidone is sometimes used to manage aggressive and other challenging behaviour.

3. **I.** Separation anxiety disorder is associated with the fear of harm coming to a major attachment figure and persistent worry that the child will be separated from the attachment figure. This results in the refusal to separate from the major attachment figure resulting in school refusal and difficulty in separating at night. It is distinguished from normal separation anxiety by the severity and persistence beyond the normal age (3 years).

4. **G.** OCD in childhood is more common in boys but has an equal gender distribution in adolescence. It is associated with Tourette's syndrome and pervasive developmental disorders.

5. **H.** Oppositional defiant disorder is the presence of markedly defiant or disobedient behaviour without the presence of aggressive behaviour or violation of societal norms. It occurs in one setting (e.g. home, school) and may lead to social isolation and substance misuse in the future.

- Conduct disorder would usually present with persistent behavioural problems across all settings and no respect for any societal norms.

Notes

- Asperger's syndrome is an autistic spectrum disorder characterised by an impairment in social interaction, repetitive behaviour, and restricted interests. IQ and language abilities are normal. It is more common in males.

Psychiatric disorders in children II

1. **H.** Gilles de la Tourette's syndrome occurs more commonly in boys. Male to female ratio is 3:1. The mean age of onset is 7 years. Dysregulation of the dopamine system is implicated. Motor tics usually present before vocal tics. Facial tics are often the initial symptoms. The shouting of obscenities is called coprolalia. Comorbidity with OCD and hyperkinetic disorder is common. Management includes psychoeducation, cognitive behavioural therapy, and haloperidol.

2. **G.** Enuresis is the voluntary or involuntary voiding of urine, usually at night. It is more common in boys. There is often a family history of enuresis. The age of onset should be at least 5 years of age. Primary enuresis occurs when continence was never achieved and secondary enuresis if the child was previously continent. It is important to exclude a urinary tract infection or neurological problems. Management involves the restriction of fluids before bedtime, behavioural approaches such as star charts, and using the bell and pad. Desmopressin (ADH analogue) and tricyclic drugs such as imipramine can also be used but have a higher rate of relapse compared to behavioural approaches.

3. **E.** Elective mutism is characterised by the consistent failure of the child to speak in specific social situations, such as school, despite speaking in other situations (e.g. home). Language and comprehension are normal for the child's age. The disorder occurs in early childhood and has an equal frequency in boys and girls. It is associated with a personal and family history of social anxiety.

4. **F.** Encopresis is the repeated voluntary or involuntary passage of faeces in inappropriate places in a child aged 4 or more years. It is more common in boys than girls. Physical causes such as an anal fissure, constipation, or neurological disorders must always be excluded. Treatment aims to restore normal bowel habit. Parents are taught to minimise the shame associated with soiling (avoid punishment of the child) and behavioural methods such as star charts may help.

5. **D.** Conduct disorder is a repetitive and persistent pattern of behaviour, which results in the violation of the rights of others or of age appropriate societal norms or rules. It is more common in boys. Risk factors for the development of conduct disorder include a family history of antisocial behaviour or substance misuse, harsh inconsistent parenting, large family size, low socio-economic status, and parental criminality. About a third of patients go on to develop antisocial personality disorder in adulthood.

Notes
- Personality disorders are diagnosed in adulthood, when the individual reaches full development at the age of 18 years.

- Oppositional defiant disorder is the presence of markedly defiant or disobedient behaviour without the presence of aggressive behaviour or violation of societal norms. It occurs in one setting, and may lead to social isolation and substance misuse.

- Transient tic disorder has a duration of less than 12 months. Chronic tic disorder has a duration of over a year but can only be motor or vocal tics, but not both. Tourette's syndrome, on the other hand, is characterised by both motor and vocal tics.

Genetic disorders associated with learning disability

1. B. Down's syndrome is the most common genetic cause of learning disability. It is caused by trisomy 21 in 95% of cases, but other causes include Robertsonian translocations and mosaicism. Individuals who survive into their 40s usually develop Alzheimer's dementia. Known risk factors for Downs's syndrome include maternal age of 40 years or older, previous siblings with the disorder, and family history. Individuals with Down's syndrome usually have IQ of less than 50.

2. H. Prader–Willi syndrome is caused by the microdeletion of the *paternal* chromosome 15. Affected individuals usually have short stature, speech abnormalities, hyperorality, hypogonadism, and mild to moderate learning disability. Associated physical features include almond-shaped eyes, incurved feet, and congenital hip dislocation.

- Angelman syndrome results from *maternal* deletion on chromosome 15 and is characterised by jerky limb movements, episodes of laughter, lack of speech development, epilepsy, and severe to profound learning disability.

3. J. Tuberous sclerosis is an autosomal dominant condition affecting roughly one in every 100,000 individuals. Physical features include shagreen patches (flesh coloured patches in the lumbosacral area), periungal fibromas, white macules (ash leaf-shaped hypopigmented areas), retinal phakomas, and adenoma sabaceum. Learning disability occurs in 60–70%, usually of a severe nature. Patients may also present with autism, hyperkinetic disorder, severe epilepsy, kidney problems, and schizophrenia.

4. G. Phenylketonuria is an autosomal recessive condition caused by a deficiency of the phenylalanine hydroxylase enzyme. It is detected by the Guthrie test at 6–14 days after birth. This is a treatable cause of severe learning disability, but if left untreated, can lead to accumulation of phenylalanine. Along with severe learning disability, it can also manifest with hyperactivity, temper tantrums, echolalia, and neurological signs (stooped posture, tremor). Treatment is with a phenylalanine free diet.

5. D. Fragile X syndrome is caused by CGG trinucleotide repeat sequences, and has a dominant X-linked transmission. Fragile X is the second most common cause of learning disability and is characterised by large ears, long narrow face, hyperextendible fingers, mitral valve prolapse, and large testicles. Individuals may have also autism and hyperkinetic disorder.

Notes

- Lesch–Nyhan syndrome is an X-linked recessive condition which results in hyperuricaemia. Behavioural symptoms include self-mutilation and physical aggression.

- Edward's syndrome occurs due to trisomy 18. It is associated with learning disability, craniofacial abnormalities, rocker-bottom feet, overlapping fifth and index finger, and cardiac and renal abnormalities. Most infants die within 3 months.

- Tay–Sachs disease is an autosomal recessive condition resulting from the accumulation of gangliosides in the nervous system. It is most common in Ashkenazi Jews. Individuals present with cognitive difficulties, speech difficulties, motor deficits, dysphagia, and ataxia. Psychosis is also a recognised complication.

- Galactosaemia is an autosomal recessive disorder of carbohydrate metabolism characterised by lethargy, vomiting, and jaundice in the neonatal period. It can result in mental retardation, ovarian dysfunction, and death if untreated.

Psychiatric syndromes I

1. **J.** Othello syndrome is a delusion of jealousy and the belief that one's partner is being unfaithful. The individual goes to great lengths to obtain evidence for the affair and may search the partner's underwear or bed sheets for stains. In some cases the allegations may actually be true but it is the nature of the evidence in which the allegations are based on which makes it a delusion. There is a risk of violence towards the partner or her alleged partner. Othello syndrome occurs in patients with alcohol dependency but may occur in other psychotic illnesses and in organic brain disease.

2. **F.** Ekbom's syndrome is a delusion that one's skin has become infested with insects or mites (delusion of infestation). It can occur in alcohol withdrawal, cocaine intoxication, acute confusional states, psychotic illnesses, dementia, or may be secondary to tactile hallucinations.

3. D. De Clerambault's syndrome (erotomania) is the delusion that someone, usually a male with a high social status, is in love with the patient. The patient (usually female) makes inappropriate attempts to contact him and becomes angry when her advances are rejected. She may resort to violence. This delusion may occur as part of schizophrenia or may occur alone as part of a persistent delusional disorder.

4. A. The central feature of chronic fatigue syndrome is fatigue and patients often associate the symptoms to a previous viral infection. The aetiology remains unknown. Treatment involves antidepressant therapy where there is evidence of affective symptoms and cognitive behavioural therapy with graded exercise.

5. B. Cotard's syndrome is associated with nihilistic delusions that an organ or part of the body does not exist and if severe, the patient may believe that he or she does not exist. This syndrome occurs most commonly in depression with psychotic features, particularly in the elderly.

Notes
- Syndrome of delusional misidentification is an umbrella term referring to illnesses where the patient is unable to correctly identify another person or place. Some illnesses that fall within this remit are Capgras' syndrome and Fregoli's syndrome.

- Munchausen's syndrome is a factitious disorder in which individuals intentionally produce symptoms and false histories for the primary purpose of obtaining medical treatment (to assume the sick role).

Psychiatric syndromes II
1. C. Couvade's syndrome is a conversion symptom seen in the partners of pregnant women. Symptoms mimic pregnancy symptoms and usually develop at the end of the first trimester and may increase in severity. It usually resolves spontaneously. It is not a delusion.

2. A. In Capgras syndrome, the individual is convinced that one or more people that they know have been replaced by an identical looking impostor.

3. **H.** Ganser's syndrome is a dissociative disorder comprising of psychogenic physical symptoms, approximate answers, pseudohallucinations, and clouding of consciousness. Approximate answers refer to answers to questions which are not correct but are almost correct and clearly the patient has understood the question. Ganser's syndrome is occasionally seen in organic brain disease.

4. **F.** Folie a deux is also known as an induced delusional disorder. This is the situation in which two people, who have an unusually close relationship, share a delusional belief. One individual develops a psychotic illness with the delusional belief, which becomes shared by the other, who is not actually psychotic. The individual with the psychotic illness should be treated and a period of separation will lead to resolution of the symptoms in the other individual. It occurs more commonly in women. In some situations more than one individual may share the delusional belief.

5. **G.** Fregoli's syndrome is the delusional belief that a familiar person has taken on the appearance of strangers, who have a different appearance, but they are actually the same person. Both Capgras and Fregoli syndrome are due to abnormalities in facial recognition and are delusions of misidentification. They may occur in schizophrenia, cerebral lesions affecting the posterior right hemisphere (where facial recognition occurs), affective psychotic disorders, and organic psychotic disorders.

Notes

• Pseudocyesis is the false belief that one is pregnant. It may be accompanied by abdominal distension and lumbar lordosis. It can occur in both men and women.

Culture bound syndromes

1. **E.** Koro is also known as 'genital retraction syndrome' and the affected individual believes that his penis is retracting inside his body. This syndrome is experienced more commonly in young single males in Asia and the Middle East, although it has also been described in other countries. The individual may take measures to stop the penis from retracting by using splints or

other devices. It is most likely to be due to an acute anxiety state but may also be associated with depression and schizophrenia.

2. **J.** Windigo is a disorder thought to occur in the indigenous Native American population and is characterised by the fear or belief that one has been transformed into a creature that eats human flesh. It may be preceded by preoccupation with physical symptoms such as reduced appetite and nausea. It is thought to represent a form of depressive psychosis although no cases have been recorded.

3. **A.** Amok is a disorder characterised by sudden unprovoked acts of violence, which may be preceded by a period of brooding or depression. The individual has amnesia for the event. It is thought to be a dissociative or depressive disorder, and is most commonly seen in males of South Asian, African, and New Guinean descent.

4. **G.** Pibliotoq is also known as 'arctic hysteria' and has been described in females of polar Inuit origin. It is characterised by a period of excitement or impulsive acts such as tearing one's clothes off, screaming and shouting, and running out into the snow. This may be followed by seizures and coma. It is thought to be an acute dissociative state.

5. **F.** Latah has been described in Malaysian females and occurs following an experience of trauma. There is an exaggerated startle reaction, which may be accompanied by echolalia, echopraxia, and a trance-like state. It may represent an acute psychotic disorder or a dissociative disorder.

Notes

- Dhat has been described in men in the Indian subcontinent and refers to the belief that semen is being passed in urine. It is associated with lethargy, anxiety, hypochondriasis, and sexual dysfunction.

- Brain fag has been described in African students, usually at times of stress such as examinations. The individual complains of poor concentration and memory, headaches, and other somatic symptoms. It is likely to represent anxiety or depression.

- Susto is thought to occur in Central and South America following a stressful event. There is fear and anxiety associated with the belief that the soul had been stolen from the body.

- Ataque de nervios has been described in South America and occurs following a stressor. There is a trance-like state, symptoms of anxiety, impulsiveness, and depression. It is thought to be a dissociative disorder.

- Taijin kyofusho occurs in Japan and is the fear of embarrassing others with one's appearance (body odour) or behaviour. It is thought to represent social phobia.

CHAPTER 5
Treatments in psychiatry

Mechanisms of drug action

A. Acetaldehyde dehydrogenase inhibitor
B. Acetyl cholinesterase inhibitor
C. Dopamine D2 receptor antagonist
D. GABA agonist
E. Histamine H1 receptor antagonist
F. NMDA receptor antagonist
G. Opiate antagonist
H. Partial dopamine D2 agonist
I. Serotonin reuptake inhibitor
J. Unknown mechanism

For each of the following drugs used in psychiatric practice, select the most likely mechanism of drug action from the above.

1. Diazepam

2. Haloperidol

3. Fluoxetine

4. Lithium

5. Disulfiram

Treatments in psychiatry I

A. Amitriptyline
B. Buprenorphine
C. Citalopram
D. Clozapine
E. Diazepam
F. Haloperidol
G. Lithium
H. Moclobemide
I. Olanzapine
J. Procyclidine

The following patients are about to be commenced on a pharmacological treatment by their team. Select the most appropriate medication from the above that is best indicated in the given clinical presentations.

1. A 23-year-old male with no previous psychiatric history presents to hospital complaining that his neighbours have been plotting an attack on him. He also mentions that he can hear his neighbours discussing his actions and appearances all the time. He is suspicious all the time and believes that he is under surveillance by hidden cameras. The doctor prescribes this medication, but warns the patient of possible drowsiness and obesity.

2. A 28-year-old female with no previous psychiatric history presents with low mood, decreased energy, disrupted sleep, poor self-esteem, and feelings of worthlessness. She is not actively suicidal, although she remains somewhat vague about her future intentions. The treating doctor is worried about future overdoses, and decides to prescribe this medication for her mood.

3. A 45-year-old male patient with a psychotic illness has been unsettled on the ward with increasing signs of agitation. His treatment is currently under review as he had developed neuroleptic malignant syndrome following the use of atypical antipsychotics. He has an argument with a fellow patient and following this, starts screaming and breaking the ward windows. The team decides to treat this acute episode using an intramuscular combination of a short-acting benzodiazepine and this medication.

4. A 30-year-old female patient is brought to hospital by her family as she has become increasingly irritable and has not slept for a week. On the ward, she is disinhibited, emotionally labile, and hyperactive. She was admitted to hospital 8 months ago for a similar episode. The treating doctor puts her on a medication to prevent further relapses of such episodes by controlling her mood.

5. A 34-year-old male patient has been in hospital for 2 years as he remains convinced that he is of royal descent and that there is a government conspiracy to hide it. During the course of his admission, he was treated with risperidone and chlorpromazine at therapeutic doses for an adequate period of time but showed no improvement. The treating doctor prescribes a medication in an attempt to improve his mental state.

Treatments in psychiatry II

A. Acamprosate
B. Buprenorphine
C. Bupropion
D. Chlordiazepoxide
E. Disulfiram
F. Lofexidine
G. Methadone
H. Naloxone
I. Naltrexone
J. Thiamine

The following patients are about to be commenced on a pharmacological treatment by their team. Select the most appropriate medication from the above that is best indicated in the given clinical presentations.

1. A 38-year-old male with a long history of heavy alcohol use has attended a 2-week residential alcohol detoxification programme. He progresses well but is worried about the prospects of missing alcohol once he gets home as he has no support at home. At the time of discharge, therefore, he was dispensed with this medication to control his craving.

2. A 29-year-old male is admitted to hospital with a dual diagnosis of schizophrenia and heavy alcohol use. He drinks roughly 50 units of alcohol a week on average, and has been drinking heavily until the day of admission. In order to prevent withdrawal seizures from abrupt cessation of alcohol consumption on the ward, he is prescribed this medication on a stepwise sliding regimen.

3. A 23-year-old female is brought to hospital unconscious. According to the ambulance crew, she was found in the back alley unconscious with injection equipment scattered around her. On examination, she has pinpoint pupils, blood pressure of 80/47, and respiratory rate of nine per minute. The medical team gives her this medication parenterally in an attempt to reverse the effects of the offending agent.

4. A 23-year-old female is brought to hospital unconscious. She was found in the back alley unconscious with injection equipment

around her with pinpoint pupils and decreased respiration. She was successfully treated in the Emergency Department and taken to the ward. Two days later, she becomes very agitated and develops severe nausea, diarrhoea, hypertension, body aches, and dilated pupils. She is prescribed a thick liquid medication, which she needs to take everyday supervised by a pharmacist.

5. A 30-year-old male with opiate dependence and hepatitis is admitted to a private specialist inpatient detoxification unit. He successfully completes the programme and leaves the unit. In his follow-up appointment a week later, he is prescribed a medication to maintain his abstinence and prevent relapse.

Treatments in psychiatry III

A. Amitriptyline
B. Chlorpromazine
C. Donepezil
D. Fluoxetine
E. Gingko biloba
F. Lithium
G. Methadone
H. Methylphenidate
I. Phenelzine
J. Risperidone

The following patients are about to be commenced on a pharmacological treatment by their team. Select the most appropriate medication from the above that is best indicated in the given clinical presentations.

1. A 72-year-old female is referred to clinic with a 6-month history of increasing forgetfulness, apathy, and difficulties with her activities of daily living. She has become lost on several occasions in her neighbourhood and cannot recognise the faces of her grandchildren. She scores 20/30 on the mini-mental state examination (MMSE) and her physical examination is normal. A CT scan of the brain shows marked atrophy of the cerebral cortex and dilated ventricles.

2. A 12-year-old male is disruptive in class and cannot sit still. He constantly runs around the classroom and blurts out answers to questions before the teacher has time to finish the sentence. He has marked difficulties in his concentration and cannot finish any of the tasks set by the teacher. His mother is finding it increasingly difficult to manage him at home.

3. A 33-year-old female presents with a long history of persistent preoccupation with eating and binge eating, followed by vomiting. She restricts her food intake in between episodes and sometimes starves herself. She is dissatisfied with her body and fears gaining weight. On examination, her BMI is 20. She has tried psychotherapy but feels she needs further support.

4. A 28-year-old female complains of low mood, which is worse in the evenings, but she is able to enjoy some activities. She has noticed an increase in her appetite resulting in weight gain and has also been sleeping more excessively than normal. Her husband has noticed that she is more sensitive to criticism and rejection.

5. An 8-year-old male with a diagnosis of autism is frequently irritable and physically aggressive towards his mother and siblings. His parents have been using behavioural therapy as a way of reinforcing positive behaviour and although this has helped, his behaviour continues to be challenging.

Treatments in psychiatry IV

A. Behavioural therapy
B. Cognitive behavioural therapy
C. Counselling
D. Electroconvulsive therapy
E. Eye movement desensitisation and reprocessing
F. Harm reduction advice
G. Hypnotherapy
H. Psychodynamic psychotherapy
I. Social skills training
J. Twelve-step programme

The following patients require a non-pharmacological intervention for their mental health problems. Select the most appropriate treatment from the above that is best indicated or described in the following scenarios.

1. A 40-year-old male presents to a walk-in service saying that he wants treatment for his abscess on his thigh. He has a history of polysubstance abuse and has been injecting heroin regularly for the last 3 months. He does not want to stop using drugs but the clinician is concerned about the effects of his risky drug-taking behaviours on his physical health.

2. A 26-year-old male has been feeling low because he has recently lost his job and relationship due to his increasing alcohol intake. He acknowledges that he needs to control his drinking and eventually manages to stop it. In order to maintain his abstinence, he joins a therapeutic group to maintain his sobriety by sharing his personal alcohol experiences.

3. A 32-year-old female is seeing a therapist for her depression and constant feelings of inadequacy. During the sessions, they explore why she feels inadequate and discovers that she always compares herself to the very best and deliberately sets high standards for herself. They then work on methods to stop her from comparing herself to others in order to prevent her from feeling low.

4. A 63-year-old male with a long history of severe depression is admitted to hospital because he has not been eating or drinking

for several days. He claims that he does not see the point in eating because his 'death is around the corner'. This current episode was brought on despite him being on adequate medications including antidepressants. Clinically he shows signs of dehydration and appears emaciated.

5. A 30-year-old female is admitted to hospital in a severely agitated state, complaining of being anxious and not being able to sleep or concentrate for a few days. This appears to be triggered by disturbing images and nightmares of an attempted rape she experienced 2 weeks ago. The treating doctor decides to refer her for a therapy specifically aimed for her condition to reduce her anxiety with these disturbing thoughts.

Side effects of psychiatric medications I

A. Amitriptyline
B. Clozapine
C. Diazepam
D. Fluoxetine
E. Lithium
F. Methadone
G. Olanzapine
H. Phenelzine
I. Sodium valproate
J. Venlafaxine

The following patients are currently on medication for a psychiatric problem. Select the most appropriate drug from the above that is implicated or responsible for each of the following adverse/side effects.

1. A 22-year-old female is recently commenced on a medication and shortly after develops nausea, diarrhoea, headache, insomnia, and increased anxiety. She also complains of decreased libido and anorgasmia.

2. A 50-year-old male is commenced on a medication and develops dry mouth, blurred vision, drowsiness, and palpitations. On examination, he is hypotensive and his ECG reveals mild QT prolongation.

3. A 45-year-old female is commenced on a medication by her psychiatrist. She subsequently presents to hospital after experiencing severe headaches and blurred vision at home. Her physical examination is remarkable for a raised blood pressure of 196/110. On assessment, she reveals that she had some red wine and pickled herring at a restaurant.

4. A 42-year-old female has been stable on her medication regimen for the last few months. However, she is urgently brought to hospital by her husband for slurred speech, ataxia, and confusion. According to the husband, his wife was recently commenced on a diuretic for hypertension and following this complained of diarrhoea, vomiting, and a coarse tremor.

5. A 33-year-old male was commenced on a medication for his psychiatric problems on the ward. A few days later, he complains to the ward doctor about a sore throat and lethargy. His physical examination is significant for pyrexia and his blood test shows leucocytosis and eosinophilia.

Side effects of psychiatric medications II

A. Acute dystonic reaction
B. Akathisia
C. Antipsychotic-induced hyperprolactinaemia
D. Cheese reaction
E. Malignant hyperthermia
F. Neuroleptic malignant syndrome
G. Parkinsonism
H. Serotonin syndrome
I. Tardive dyskinesia
J. Wernicke–Korsakoff syndrome

Select the most appropriate item from the above that best fits with the given clinical descriptions.

1. A 35-year-old male with a first psychotic episode was commenced on haloperidol. Few days later, he was noted to be pacing constantly and was unable to sit still. When questioned by a nurse, he reports feeling edgy and restless.

2. A 35-year-old male with a first psychotic episode was commenced on haloperidol. Few days later, he was noted to be arching his back with eyes rolled backwards. He was given an anticholinergic medication and the symptom eventually subsided.

3. A 35-year-old male with a first psychotic episode was commenced on haloperidol. Few hours later, he developed a fever and was noted to be rigid. His vital observations were measured by the nurse and showed a temperature of 39°C, respiratory rate of 38 breaths per minute, pulse of 110, and a blood pressure of 180/104 mmHg. The on-call doctor ordered a blood test and found a raised creatinine kinase.

4. A 35-year-old male with a first psychotic episode was commenced on haloperidol. Few months later, his wife noticed that he was constantly smacking his lips and sticking his tongue out. It also seemed as if he was constantly chewing something. The wife noted that this disappeared while he was asleep.

5. A 35-year-old male with a first psychotic episode was commenced on haloperidol. As his psychotic episode was found to

be associated with severe depression, he was also commenced on an antidepressant. The patient went on weekend leave and took his medication, as well as St John's Wort which he bought at the local store. On returning to the ward, he was noted to be agitated, confused, and shivering. On examination, his temperature was 38°C and clinical examination was remarkable for myoclonus and hyperreflexia.

Psychotherapy concepts

A. Acting out
B. Countertransference
C. Denial
D. Free association
E. Projection
F. Reaction formation
G. Repression
H. Resistance
I. Splitting
J. Transference

Select the most appropriate psychotherapy concept from the above that best depicts the following clinical scenarios.

1. A 30-year-old female is undergoing psychotherapy to explore the trauma of her early childhood abuse. The psychotherapist becomes angry with the patient who arrives 30 minutes late for each session. When exploring these feelings further she realises that the patient reminds her of her own daughter who does not appreciate her.

2. A 30-year-old female is attending psychotherapy to explore the trauma of her early childhood abuse. She is unable to recall any memories of the abuse even though her mother informed her that she was abused at the age of 8 years by her uncle.

3. A 30-year-old female is attending psychotherapy to explore the trauma of her early childhood abuse. The patient is either late to most of her sessions or does not turn up to the sessions at all. The therapist explores possible reasons for this behaviour and interprets that she may be avoiding the sessions as a way of preventing painful memories about the abuse resurfacing.

4. A 30-year-old female is attending psychotherapy to explore the trauma of her early childhood abuse. Towards the end of one of her sessions, she becomes angry with the male therapist and threatens to assault him. She eventually calms down and the therapist explores the possibility that he may remind her of her own father who abused her as a child.

5. A 30-year-old female is attending psychotherapy to explore the trauma of her early childhood abuse. During the therapy she tells the therapist how wonderful and understanding he is and that the previous therapist she had was incompetent.

Answers

Mechanism of drug action

1. **D.** Diazepam is a benzodiazepine and acts as a modulator on GABA receptors. Benzodiazepines are relatively safe in overdoses and have a number of different uses. They are used in the treatment of anxiety disorders, agitation, insomnia, alcohol withdrawal symptoms, epilepsy, and as muscle relaxants. Side effects include sedation, ataxia, confusion, respiratory depression, and psychological and physical dependency.

2. **C.** Haloperidol is a typical antipsychotic drug. All antipsychotic drugs exert their antipsychotic effects through blockade of the dopamine D2 receptor. Typical antipsychotic drugs are more likely to be associated with extrapyramidal side effects such as parkinsonism, acute dystonic reactions, akathisia, and tardive dyskinesia. Atypical drugs are usually tolerated better but can cause weight gain and predispose patients to diabetes mellitus.

3. **I.** Fluoxetine is a selective serotonin reuptake inhibitor. They are used in the treatment of depression and anxiety disorders such as obsessive-compulsive disorder, post-traumatic stress disorder, and panic disorder. They are usually tolerated better than tricyclic antidepressants. Side effects include gastrointestinal effects, headaches, insomnia, and agitation.

4. **J.** The mechanism of action of lithium is unknown, but it is thought to affect secondary messenger systems within the cell, including inhibition of cyclic AMP. Lithium is most commonly used in the treatment of mania and prophylaxis of bipolar affective disorder.

5. **A.** Disulfiram is used in the maintenance treatment of patients with alcohol dependency to maintain abstinence. It is an acetaldehyde dehydrogenase inhibitor and thus those who drink alcohol while taking the drug will experience unpleasant effects such as nausea, vomiting, and flushing due to the build up of acetaldehyde. It is aimed at discouraging people from drinking but requires a lot of motivation.

Notes

• Acetyl cholinesterase inhibitors are used in the treatment of Alzheimer's disease and include drugs like donepezil. Side effects of these drugs include nausea, vomiting, diarrhoea, insomnia, and weakness.

• Partial dopamine D2 agonism is the underlying mechanism for aripiprazole, which is a new atypical antipsychotic drug used in the treatment of schizophrenia and mania. It is well tolerated and does not seem to be associated with hyperprolactinaemia, impaired glucose tolerance, or significant weight gain commonly seen with atypicals.

• Blockade of histamine H1 receptor leads to sedation, anxiolysis, and weight gain.

Treatment in psychiatry I

1. **I.** Atypical drugs such as olanzapine and risperidone should be used first line in the treatment of schizophrenia, according to the UK National Institute for Health and Clinical Excellence (NICE) guidelines. Atypical drugs are less likely to cause movement disorders (such as parkinsonism and dyskinesia) and may be better at reducing the negative symptoms of schizophrenia, although they can be associated with other side effects such as obesity, diabetes, and hyperprolactinaemia.

2. **C.** Selective serotonin reuptake inhibitors such as citalopram and fluoxetine are recommended in the first-line treatment of depression as they tend to be tolerated better than tricyclics (such as amitriptyline).
   • Amitriptyline (and other tricyclics) is associated with a decrease in cardiac conduction and lower seizure threshold. They are also known to be toxic in overdose, and thus are not recommended in those who may take an overdose.

3. **F.** In employing rapid tranquillisation techniques, the most common combination is that of a short-acting benzodiazepine (usually lorazepam 2 mg) with an antipsychotic (usually haloperidol 10 mg). The antipsychotic administered can be typical (e.g. haloperidol) or atypical (e.g. olanzapine), but as the patient has previously developed a bad reaction to atypicals in this scenario, haloperidol should be given.

4. **G.** Lithium is a mood stabiliser used in treating affective disorders such as bipolar affective disorder and schizoaffective disorder. They are employed mainly as prophylaxis against mania, although they are also used as augmentation therapy in treatment-resistant depression.

5. **D.** Clozapine is indicated in treatment-resistant schizophrenia, defined as a lack of response to treatment with two antipsychotics (one being an atypical). Although it is a highly efficacious drug ('gold standard'), it is associated with serious adverse effects such as agranulocytosis and thus requires regular blood tests.

Notes

• Diazepam is a benzodiazepine used as an anxiolytic or sedative.

• Moclobemide is a monoamine oxidase inhibitor (MAOI) used in the treatment of atypical depression (depression presenting with features such as hypersomnia and hyperphagia). Although other MAOIs irreversibly inhibit monoamine oxidase, the effects of moclobemide are reversible. The major side effects of MAOIs are hypertensive crisis on ingestion of tyramine (cheese reaction), antimuscarinic effects (dry mouth, blurred vision), and hepatotoxicity.

• Procyclidine is an anticholinergic agent used in the treatment of drug-induced extrapyramidal side effects (parkinsonism, dyskinesia, akathisia), commonly resulting from administration of haloperidol or other typical antipsychotics.

Treatments in psychiatry II

1. **A.** Acamprosate is thought to act by enhancing GABA transmission in the brain by blocking the NMDA glutamate receptors, with the aim of reducing alcohol cravings. There is evidence from a randomised controlled trial to suggest that acamprosate can increase the rates of abstinence and double the time to relapse. It should be discontinued if the patient returns to regular drinking. Unlike disulfiram it is not associated with an aversive reaction if taken with alcohol.

2. **D.** Chlordiazepoxide is given to relieve alcohol withdrawal symptoms and to prevent alcohol withdrawal seizures. Most patients wishing to undergo detoxification can be given support to complete this in the community. Inpatient detoxification is

recommended where there is a history of withdrawal seizures, symptoms of Wernicke–Korsakoff syndrome, comorbid mental illness, physical illness, suicidal ideation, failure of outpatient detoxification, or lack of a stable environment at home.

3. **H.** Naloxone is a competitive antagonist of the mu-opioid receptor and is used as an antidote in the treatment of opiate overdose, which left untreated, may lead to respiratory depression. It has a short half-life and therefore must be given repeatedly. The patient in this scenario is clearly showing signs of opiate overdose, which needs to be treated urgently.

4. **G.** Methadone is a synthetic opioid used in substitute prescribing for opiate-dependent patients who are going through withdrawal. It is a long-acting synthetic opioid suitable for daily dosing, usually prescribed daily and supervised by a pharmacist.

5. **I.** Naltrexone is a competitive antagonist at the kappa- and mu-opioid receptors used as an aid in remaining abstinent from opiates by blocking opiate intake. It can also be used to facilitate rapid detoxification from opiates in specialist inpatient facilities. In alcohol dependency, it reduces the 'highs' associated with drinking.

Notes

• Buprenorphine is a partial opiate agonist licensed for the treatment of opiate dependence in substitute prescribing, similar to methadone. However, it is thought to produce less euphoria than methadone at higher doses and can be given once every 2 or 3 days. It is usually taken as a tablet sublingually.

• Buproprion (zyban) is a noradrenaline and dopamine reuptake inhibitor used in depression, nicotine cessation, and occasionally in attention deficit hyperactivity disorder.

• Disulfiram (antabuse) blocks the pathway by which alcohol is broken down by the enzyme acetaldehyde dehydrogenase, resulting in the build-up of acetaldehyde with alcohol consumption. This leads to unpleasant effects such as flushing, nausea, and headaches and the aim is to associate drinking alcohol with these effects. Disulfiram should only be started once patients are abstinent from alcohol and its use should be supervised at home by family or friends.

- Thiamine (vitamin B1) is given to patients who abuse alcohol in order to treat Wernicke's encepahalopathy or prevents its occurrence.

- Lofexidine is an alpha-adrenergic agonist used to minimise opiate withdrawal symptoms such as sweating and lacrimation. It can cause hypotension, and thus blood pressure needs to be monitored when starting a patient on the drug.

Treatments in psychiatry III

1. **C.** The patient has moderate Alzheimer's dementia, and thus treatment with an acetylcholinesterase inhibitor such as donepezil is recommended. The most recent UK National Institute of Clinical Excellence (NICE) guidelines recommend that acetylcholinesterase inhibitors should only be prescribed in people with moderate dementia with an MMSE score between 10 and 20. The diagnosis should be made by specialists and only specialists should initiate treatment. Assessments need to be carried out 2–4 months after initiation and then every 6 months, including an assessment of activities of daily living, MMSE, and carers' opinion. Treatment should only continue if there is an improvement or no deterioration.

2. **H.** Methylphenidate (ritalin) is a psychostimulant used in the first-line treatment of hyperkinetic disorder, as recommended by the UK NICE guidelines. Although the exact mechanism of action is not fully understood, the paradoxical effect of a stimulant is thought to have some effect in increasing concentration and decreasing impulsivity. Side effects of methylphenidate include insomnia, decreased appetite and weight loss, dysphoria, hypertension, worsening of tics, and a slight growth suppression.
   - Other stimulants that are used to treat hyperkinetic disorder include dexamphetamine and pemoline.
   - Behavioural management includes parental training, where parents are encouraged to reward desired behaviour and to pay less attention to undesirable behaviour.

3. **D.** There is some evidence to suggest that high doses of fluoxetine are associated with reduced frequency of binge eating and vomiting in patients with bulimia nervosa. However, the primary treatment should be psychotherapy.

4. **I.** The patient is displaying features of atypical depression, for which monoamine oxidase inhibitors such as phenelzine are considered to be more effective than other antidepressants.

5. **J.** Risperidone is sometimes used in the management of hyperactivity, aggression, and repetitive behaviours in children with autism. However, it is advisable to try psychological treatments such as behavioural therapy and family therapy in the first instance.

Notes

*   Gingko biloba is a herbal remedy used as a cognitive enhancer and there is some evidence to suggest that it may be effective in mild to moderate Alzheimer's dementia. However, it is not widely used in the UK.

Treatments in psychiatry IV

1. **F.** Harm reduction advice involves advising patients about the harmful effects of drugs and providing education about the ways in which risks associated with its use can be minimised. It is particularly useful in opiate users who have no desire to give up injecting, and include giving advice on where to obtain clean needles and free condoms, and offering regular screening for blood-borne viruses.

2. **J.** Twelve-step programmes uphold 12 core principles in aiding recovery from addictions and the most prominent example is Alcoholics Anonymous (AA). As part of the 12 steps, individuals must admit that their lives have become powerless as a result of drinking, and that there is a higher power that they must turn to for help.

3. **B.** Cognitive behavioural therapy is a short, collaborative therapy with the aim of relieving symptoms and developing new skills. It looks at the way in which thoughts, actions, and biological responses are interrelated and aims to intervene in this relationship to bring forth a change in behaviour. It was developed by Beck in the 1960s, after observing that many of his depressed patients held strong negative views of themselves, the world, and the future (Beck's cognitive triad).

4. D. Electroconvulsive therapy (ECT) is a treatment involving the induction of medically controlled seizures through the placement of electrodes on the temporal region. ECT is typically given two to three times a week for up to 12 sessions. According to the UK National Institute for Health and Clinical Excellence guidelines (2003), ECT is indicated for the treatment of severe depression, catatonia, or prolonged mania. The aim is to achieve rapid and short-term relief of severe symptoms only after other treatments have been inadequate, unless it is a life-threatening condition. Notable side effects are short-term memory loss, headaches, and anaesthetic complications.

5. E. Eye movement desensitisation and reprocessing (EMDR) uses voluntary multi-saccadic eye movements to reduce anxiety associated with disturbing thoughts. It has been shown to be useful in the treatment of post-traumatic stress disorder. It was developed by Francine Shapiro in 1987, when she realised that moving her eyes relieved her from her own personal traumatic memories.

Notes

- Behavioural therapy aims to bring forth behavioural change through specific techniques such as exposure and response prevention, systemic desensitisation, and flooding.

- Counselling in psychotherapeutic terms refers to a broader range of therapies that incorporate listening, release of emotion, restoration of morale, advice, and guidance. It is usually patient centred and can be given in a variety of settings.

- Psychodynamic psychotherapy attaches great importance to relationships, in particular the therapeutic relationship formed between the therapist and the patient. It looks at previous relationships, conflicts, and experiences to assess their impact on current functioning. The therapist and the patient meet roughly once a week for up to a year.

- Social skills training aims to improve social behaviour, which can be improved through modelling, guided practice, and role play. Examples include assertiveness training and anger management.

Side effects of psychiatric medications I

1. **D.** Fluoxetine is a selective serotonin reuptake inhibitor and associated with side effects such as nausea, diarrhoea, sexual dysfunctions, insomnia, and agitation on commencing.

2. **A.** Amitriptyline is a tricyclic antidepressant and blocks a wide range of receptors including muscarinic (dry mouth, constipation, blurring of vision), H1 histaminergic (weight gain, drowsiness), and adrenergic (hypotension, sexual dysfunction). Cardiotoxic effects include arrhythmias, ventricular tachycardias, and QT prolongation. Contraindications for the use of these drugs include a recent myocardial infarction, prostatic hypertrophy, and narrow-angle glaucoma.

3. **H.** Phenelzine is a monoamine oxidase inhibitor (MAOI) used in the treatment of depression, usually with atypical features. Hypertensive crisis ('cheese reaction') is associated with consumption of products containing tyramine such as cheese, fava been, red wine, and liver. Tyramine is normally broken down by monoamine oxidase but inhibition of this enzyme results in accumulation. Other side effects of MAOI include anticholinergic effects, postural hypotension, insomnia, ankle oedema, and paraesthesia. Moclobemide is a reversible MAOI and is less likely to cause hypertensive reactions.

4. **E.** The patient in this vignette developed lithium toxicity as a result of diuretic usage. Lithium toxicity occurs when the level of serum lithium exceeds 2 mmol/L, although signs can start appearing at lower doses, especially in elderly patients. Signs and symptoms include increased tremor, anorexia, nausea, lethargy, restlessness, and increased tone. This may progress to ataxia, dysarthria, confusion, coma, and even death. Since lithium is excreted by the kidneys, anything that reduces renal clearance of lithium can lead to increased serum levels, including non-steroidal anti-inflammatory drugs (NSAIDs). Dehydration and diuretics can also raise serum lithium concentration. The usual serum target for lithium is between 0.4 and 1.0 mmol/L. Early side effects of lithium include a dry mouth, thirst, metallic taste to the mouth, nausea, vomiting, and a mild tremor. Long-term use lead to hypothyroidism and nephrogenic diabetes insipidus, and

therefore both thyroid and kidney functions need to be monitored regularly.

5. **B.** Agranulocytosis is one of the serious side effects of clozapine and occurs in 1% of patients. As a result, all patients must have a weekly blood test (full blood count) for the first 18 weeks, then every 2 weeks until 12 months, followed by monthly blood tests thereafter. Each patient is registered with the Clozaril Patient Monitoring Service (CPMS), which ensures that prescriptions are only given if there is a normal blood result.

Notes
- Sodium valproate is a mood stabiliser used in the treatment of acute mania and prophylaxis of bipolar affective disorder. Adverse effects include hyperammonaemia, gastric irritation, hair loss, hepatic failure, pancreatitis, and thrombocytopaenia.

- Venlafaxine is a serotonin and noradrenaline reuptake inhibitor (SNRI) used in treating depression. In higher doses, venlafaxine can lead to hypertension.

Side effects of psychiatric medications II
1. **B.** Akathisia is an unpleasant and distressing side effect of antipsychotic medication and is characterised by a sense of inner restlessness and an inability to stand, sit, or lie still. It may be confused with agitation or worsening of psychiatric symptoms. Treatment involves reducing the dose, switching to a less potent antipsychotic drug, and if symptoms persist, a beta-blocker such as propranolol or a benzodiazepine such as diazepam may be helpful.

2. **A.** Acute dystonias are painful sustained muscular spasms. Dystonias affecting the neck, jaw, and tongue are the most common but oculogyric crisis (eyes rolled back) and opisthotonus (arched body) may occur. It may be mistaken for bizarre behaviour. Treatment involves discontinuation of the antipsychotic agent and emergency intramuscular treatment with an anticholinergic agent such as procyclidine.

3. **F.** Neuroleptic malignant syndrome is a rare, idiosyncratic, life-threatening reaction to antipsychotics. Symptoms include fever,

muscular rigidity, confusion, diaphoresis, tachycardia, and an unstable blood pressure. It is associated with a raised white cell count and creatinine kinase. Complications include rhabdomyolysis, renal failure, seizures, and respiratory failure. Management is supportive and involves stopping the causative antipsychotic, emergency transfer of the patient to the medical intensive care unit, oxygen, intravenous fluids, cooling blankets to decrease temperature, sodium dantrolene to reduce muscular rigidity, and benzodiazepines. In treatment-resistant cases ECT may be required.

4. I. Tardive dyskinesia is characterised by repetitive involuntary purposeless movements of the body and most commonly affects the perioral region (lips, tongue, jaw). It is more common in females (especially the elderly) and those who have been on long-term antipsychotics. It is *exacerbated* by anticholinergic drugs. Management involves reducing the dose of the antipsychotic drug, withdrawal of anticholinergic drugs, and if symptoms are severe, tetrabenazine or benzodiazepines such as clonazepam can be used. Clozapine may be used in cases that have failed to respond to these measures.

5. H. Serotonin syndrome is a rare syndrome that may occur following the initiation or increase in the dose of a serotonergic agent such as an antidepressant. It is more likely to occur when a combination of serotonergic agents are used (e.g. antidepressants and St John's Wort). Typical symptoms and signs include agitation, confusion, tremor, sweating, diarrhoea, fever, myoclonus, and hyperreflexia. Management is supportive and involves immediate transfer to the medical ward (if severe), intravenous fluids, reduction of temperature with cooling blankets and ice packs, and benzodiazepines to treat agitation and myoclonus.

Notes
- Malignant hyperthermia is a rare genetic condition that mimics neuroleptic malignant syndrome. It is associated with exposure to inhaled anaesthetics and is characterised by muscular rigidity and increased body temperature.

- Extrapyramidal side effects (parkinsonism, tardive dyskinesia, acute dystonic reaction, akathisia) and hyperprolactinaemia are well-known side effects of antipsychotics.

Psychotherapy concepts

1. **B.** Countertransference is the unconscious re-experiencing of feelings associated with important figures in the therapist's life in the current relationship with the patient.

2. **G.** Repression is a defence mechanism that pushes away unpleasant feelings, thoughts, and memories into the unconscious. It forms the basis for other defence mechanisms.

3. **H.** Resistance refers to methods used by the patient consciously or unconsciously to prevent an intervention designed to help him or her from working, for example turning up to therapy sessions late, concealing vital information, or terminating it altogether. This may result from the patient's desire to avoid painful memories (repression resistance) or to form a therapeutic relationship with the therapist (transference resistance).

4. **J.** Transference represents the re-experiencing of emotions and thoughts that are associated with a significant person in the patient's life in the current relationship with the therapist. Examination of both transference and countertransference is an important component of the therapy.

5. **I.** Splitting is a defence mechanism that categorises people (or even the same person at different times) as either all-good or all-bad in order to avoid ambivalent feelings. This is commonly used by individuals with borderline personality disorder.

Notes

- Therapeutic alliance is the working relationship between the patient and the therapist, and is the foundation of all successful psychotherapeutic treatments.

- Free association involves the patient revealing everything that comes into the mind no matter how embarrassing it may be. It is the main route for the exploration of the unconscious.

- Acting out is the avoidance of unacceptable feelings by behaving in an inappropriate or attention seeking manner.

- Defence mechanisms are unconscious mental processes that are used by the ego to keep conflicts out of awareness and therefore reduce anxiety.
  - Denial involves denying the external reality of an unpleasant experience or memory from entering one's own conscious mind. This is an active, conscious process and the individual's denial is usually obvious to another person.
  - Projection is used by patients who have paranoid symptoms and is the attribution of one's unacceptable thoughts or feelings on to others.
  - Reaction formation is behaving or feeling in a way that is opposite to one's unacceptable instinctual impulses, for example a man angry at his wife acting extra nice to her.

CHAPTER 6

Management issues in psychiatry

Psychiatric management

A. Call the police
B. Containment in seclusion
C. Depot antipsychotic medication
D. Mental Health Act assessment and placement on Section 5(2)
E. Mental Health Act assessment and placement on Section 5(4)
F. Patient completes "discharge against medical advice" form
G. Rapid tranquillisation with intramuscular medication
H. Rapid tranquillisation with oral medication
I. Referral to Psychiatric Intensive Care Unit (PICU)
J. No further action required.

Select the most appropriate next line of management from the above for each of the following scenarios.

1. A 23-year-old female is admitted voluntarily to the ward following an overdose. While on the ward, her behaviour becomes erratic and she demands that she no longer wants to remain on the ward. The duty doctor assesses her mental state and elicits auditory hallucinations telling her to kill herself.

2. A 20-year-old male with a known history of schizophrenia is admitted to the ward compulsorily following deterioration of his mental state. One day while out on unescorted community leave, he returns to the ward agitated and distressed, and discloses that he had consumed cannabis. He becomes irritable and starts shouting abuse at the nurses when they request a urine sample for a drug screen. The nurse attempts to 'talk him down' but this fails.

3. A 23-year-old male is referred to a psychiatric outpatient clinic by his doctor. While waiting for the doctor, he informs the receptionist that he has a gun in his possession and plans to shoot his wife when he returns home as he has discovered that she has been cheating on him with the next door neighbour.

4. A 29-year-old male who is detained compulsorily in hospital has been difficult to manage due to his persistent threatening behaviour towards staff and other patients. He has also absconded from the ward on two occasions and was brought back by the police. Despite efforts to engage with the patient, he locks himself up in his room claiming that he no longer wants any help.

5. A 31-year-old male admitted compulsorily with a manic episode becomes increasingly disturbed on the ward. Despite being prescribed olanzapine and lithium by his psychiatrist, he refuses to take them and regularly requires intramuscular medication of lorazepam and haloperidol to 'calm him down'.

1983 Mental Health Act I

A. Section 2
B. Section 3
C. Section 4
D. Section 5(2)
E. Section 5(4)
F. Section 17
G. Section 37/41
H. Section 117
I. Section 135
J. Section 136

Select the most appropriate section of the 1983 Mental Health Act of England and Wales from the above that is best indicated or depicted in the following scenarios.

1. A 24-year-old male is reported to the police by railway staff who stopped him from attempting to jump in front of a train. The police subsequently take him to the nearest hospital Emergency Department for assessment.

2. A 28-year-old male was detained in hospital compulsorily due to relapse of his psychotic illness. His mental state rapidly improves while in hospital and he is due for discharge in a few days. A multidisciplinary discharge planning meeting is organised for him under this section to ensure that he receives appropriate care and follow up after leaving the hospital, including allocation of a care coordinator and regular attendance in outpatient's clinic.

3. A 25-year-old male is brought to the hospital Emergency Department by his mother who is worried about her personal safety after he attempted to strangle her while she was sleeping. He admits to hearing voices telling him to harm his mother as he believes that she is the devil in disguise. He has no previous psychiatric history and refuses to be admitted to hospital.

4. A 32-year-old female who was admitted voluntarily to a psychiatric ward with depression is requesting to leave. The nursing staff are concerned about her safety as she has been expressing the desire to end her life. The duty doctor is unavailable as she is assessing another patient in the hospital Emergency Department.

5. A 36-year-old male is taken to see his family doctor by his wife after he was found trying to hang himself. The man refuses psychiatric help, but the doctor is concerned about the high risk of suicide and wants to arrange an urgent admission to psychiatric hospital. The approved social worker arrives for assessment but no other doctor was available.

1983 Mental Health Act II

A. Section 2
B. Section 3
C. Section 4
D. Section 5(2)
E. Section 5(4)
F. Section 17
G. Section 37/41
H. Section 117
I. Section 135
J. Section 136

Select the most appropriate section of the 1983 Mental Health Act of England and Wales from the above that is best indicated in the following scenarios.

1. The son of a 60-year-old male is concerned that his father has been losing his memory and neglecting himself since his wife died 6 months ago. He has lost weight significantly and has accidentally left the gas on a number of occasions. His residence is in a state of squalor but he has been refusing to open the door to social services or his family doctor despite efforts to carry out a Mental Health Act assessment.

2. A 31-year-old male with a long history of bipolar affective disorder has a manic relapse after stopping his medication 3 months ago. He is dishevelled in appearance and has been wandering the streets naked, claiming that he has special powers that will heal the world. His care coordinator and psychiatrist subsequently arrange a Mental Health Act assessment as he refused to be admitted to hospital voluntarily.

3. A 44-year-old male is arrested after stabbing his mother. During the court hearing, the forensic psychiatrist reports that he was suffering from psychotic symptoms at the time of the incident and continues to experience auditory hallucinations and persecutory delusions. A recommendation is made for him to be transferred to an appropriate high-security ward for psychiatric treatment.

4. A 28-year-old female who was admitted to hospital compulsorily following a relapse of schizophrenia is requesting to go to a

church service on Sunday. She has been settled on the ward and her psychiatrist agrees that she can leave the ward if escorted by a member of staff.

5. A 32-year-old female who was admitted voluntarily to hospital following a relapse of depression is requesting to leave during the weekend. The duty doctor is called to review her and feels that she is at high risk of suicide. However, as the patient remains adamant on leaving hospital, the duty doctor places the patient on this section to prevent her from leaving hospital over the weekend.

Ethical issues in psychiatry

A. Assess capacity
B. Assess Gillick competence
C. Assess testamentary capacity
D. Break patient confidentiality
E. Child protection procedure
F. Obtain consent from carers
G. Obtain parental consent
H. Treat under Mental Capacity Act 2005
I. Treatment under the Mental Health Act
J. No further action indicated

Select the most appropriate next line of management from the above for each of the following statements.

1. A 30-year-old depressed female is brought to hospital following a large overdose of paracetamol. She has severe liver impairment and the surgeon is trying to book an urgent liver transplant for the following week but she is flatly refusing to give consent for the procedure. The surgeons have not interviewed further following this.

2. A 65-year-old male with schizophrenia who is detained compulsorily in hospital is brought to the hospital Emergency Department following a ruptured abdominal aortic aneurysm. He requires urgent surgery but refuses as he believes that the surgeons are planning to implant a device into his abdomen that will enable the government to monitor his thoughts.

3. A 13-year-old female consults her family doctor about obtaining contraception. She would like to start the oral contraceptive pill but does not want her parents to find out that she is sexually active with her 15-year-old boyfriend.

4. A 17-year-old female is admitted to hospital compulsorily under the Mental Health Act with severe anorexia nervosa and a BMI of 12. She has not eaten for several weeks and is refusing oral intake on the ward. The psychiatric team would like to feed her via a nasogastric tube but she refuses to consent to this, citing that she is too fat already.

5. A 78-year-old male with moderate Alzheimer's dementia continues to drive his car, despite his psychiatrist strongly recommending that he stops driving. He recently drove his car into a parked vehicle but fortunately no one was hurt. His wife has tried hiding the car keys in the past, but asks the psychiatrist for further support.

Professionals in psychiatry

A. Approved social worker
B. Care coordinator
C. Clinical psychologist
D. Duty doctor
E. General practitioner
F. Hospital managers
G. Mental Health Act Administrator
H. Occupational therapist
I. Registered mental nurse
J. Responsible medical officer

Select the most appropriate professional from the above that would be able to best provide the service required in the following scenarios.

1. A 19-year-old male was admitted compulsorily to hospital for a first psychotic episode. However, he disagrees with the diagnosis and wants to leave the hospital at the earliest instance. Rather than waiting for a tribunal, he applies for a hearing with a panel headed by this professional.

2. A 40-year-old male with schizophrenia is about to be discharged from hospital after a seven year hospital admission. The team is concerned about his ability to look after himself as he has been institutionalised for a long time. This professional decides to assess the patient's activities of daily living to recommend suitable accommodations.

3. A 37-year-old female admitted to hospital compulsorily with a relapse of bipolar affective disorder has improved in mental state after a 4-week treatment. She would now like to proceed with escorted leave from the hospital, and this professional completes the necessary legal paperwork.

4. A 26-year-old male was admitted to hospital compulsorily and diagnosed with schizoaffective disorder. At his discharge meeting, it was agreed that he would be put on a Care Programme Approach (CPA) to ensure that he receives the necessary mental and social care needs after discharge. This professional is the named deputy to ensure that all the aims in the CPA are followed in the community.

5. A 30-year-old male with a diagnosis of mixed anxiety and depressive disorder has become increasingly agitated and resumed drinking despite being abstinent for 3 years. He finds that the temptation of bars and his ongoing feelings of inadequacy reverts him to drinking. His local psychiatric service refers this patient to this professional to explore and modify his drinking and feelings.

Psychiatric services

A. Assertive outreach team
B. Befriending service
C. Community drug and alcohol team
D. Community mental health team
E. Crisis resolution team
F. Day hospital service
G. Early intervention service
H. Forensic service
I. Primary care team
J. Social services

Select the most appropriate service from the above that is best indicated in the management of the following scenarios.

1. A 25-year-old female who is a successful business executive is concerned that she may be drinking excessively. She drinks moderately, but on occasions consumes around 16 units of alcohol a week. Her drinking has never affected her work or social life, but she would like some advice on cutting down.

2. A 23-year-old male has been in hospital six times over the last 2 years with a manic relapse of bipolar affective disorder. These admissions have all been preceded by non-compliance to medications and disengagements from standard psychiatric services.

3. A 22-year-old medical student presents with a 6-month history of deterioration in his college work, social withdrawal, and strange beliefs that the atmosphere is contaminated with poison. He has no previous psychiatric history, and his general practitioner (GP) feels that he would merit intervention from a specialist psychiatric team rather than standard community psychiatric care.

4. A 29-year-old male was admitted to hospital for the third time and diagnosed with bipolar affective disorder. At his discharge meeting, it was agreed that his mental health will be monitored in the community by this service through outpatient clinics and standard Care Programme Approach (CPA) managed by his care coordinator.

5. A 30-year-old female presents to hospital in a tearful and agitated state claiming that she is a failure. She was recently fired from her job for a mistake that she had made. On assessment, she is not actively suicidal and indicates she wants to get better, but she remains extremely tearful and complains that she feels scared of being alone.

Answers

Psychiatric management

1. **D.** The patient is informal and is now requesting to leave the ward. Given the high risk of suicide she should be assessed under the 1983 Mental Health Act of England and Wales and placed under Section 5(2) if appropriate, which will detain the patient for up to 3 days until a formal Mental Health Act assessment takes place.

2. **H.** De-escalation should always be attempted in the first instance and this involves techniques aimed at calming the patient. However, if this is unsuccessful, then rapid tranquillisation is the next option. This is the administration of medication to calm or sedate a disturbed patient, and is offered orally in the first instance. If the patient refuses oral medication or does not respond to this, then the next step would be intramuscular medication. The principal is to reduce patient suffering, to facilitate improved communication, and to reduce the risks to the patient and others. Most commonly lorazepam (benzodiazepine) and haloperidol (antipsychotic) are used together but they may be used on their own. Once administered, patients should have their vital signs monitored due to the risk of cardiovascular collapse and respiratory depression.

3. **A.** Due to the high risk of harm to his wife and others, the police should be informed immediately to have his gun removed and taken to custody. The patient would then have his mental state assessed by a psychiatrist there to determine further course of action.

4. **I.** In this situation, the patient would be better managed in a PICU given his persistent aggression, high absconding risk, and his reluctance to engage with staff (including administration of medication at present).

5. **C.** Depot medication is useful for patients who are refusing oral antipsychotic medication or requiring regular intramuscular medication. It can be given any time from once weekly to once monthly and thus is particularly useful for those with difficulty with compliance in the community.

Notes

- Rapid tranquilisation with *intravenous* medication is a last resort in acutely disturbed/violent patients and may be used when oral and intramuscular medication has failed. It is rarely used.

• Seclusion facilities are available in PICU and used to keep a patient isolated alone for periods when their behaviours become too dangerous or risky even in a PICU setting. Patients placed in seclusion are regularly reviewed by nursing staff and psychiatrist.

1983 Mental Health Act I

1. J. Section 136 is exercised by the police to bring a person who appears to be suffering from a mental illness from a public place to a place of safety. The place of safety is usually a designated mental health setting such as the hospital Accident and Emergency Department or the police station. The section lasts for up to 72 hours, and the purpose is to enable the individual to be assessed by mental health services. The section may be converted to a Section 2 or 3 if the individual is found to have a mental disorder requiring a hospital admission (and is refusing admission), or the patient may be admitted informally to hospital or discharged if not found to have a mental disorder.

• A Section 135 is used by the police to bring a person from a private place (such as residence) to a place of safety.

2. H. Section 117 stipulates that there is a statutory duty for mental health services to provide aftercare for patients who have been discharged from a section. This is normally implemented under the Care Programme Approach (CPA) framework and involves identifying a care coordinator who will be responsible for ensuring coordination of all aspects of the patient's care. A care plan is also developed to address the patient's needs and specific targets are set. It is good practice for all patients, whether on section or not, to have a CPA meeting prior to discharge.

3. A. Section 2 is a recommendation for admission to a mental health unit for the purpose of assessment, which is valid for up to 28 days. It requires an application by the approved social worker (or nearest relative) and two medical recommendations, one of which must be made by a doctor who is approved under Section 12(2) as having special experience in the diagnosis and treatment of mental disorders. The patient can appeal against the section. Following a Section 2, an application may be made for a Section 3 for the purpose of treatment or the patient may be discharged off the section.

4. E. Section 5(4) enables a registered mental health nurse to stop a voluntary inpatient from leaving the hospital until a formal assessment by a doctor has been completed. It is valid for up to 6 hours.

5. C. Section 4 is an emergency section used to detain a patient in hospital for up to 3 days, and requires one medical recommendation and an application by one approved social worker or nearest relative. There is no right of appeal under this section. It is usually used when the situation is so urgent to the point that organising a Section 2 or 3 assessment is not practical.

Notes

- In order for a patient to be detained against their will under Section 2 or 3, the following clinical criteria need to be fulfilled:
  - Individual must be suffering from a mental disorder of a degree and nature that warrants treatment in a hospital, and that such treatment cannot be provided without detention.
  - Individual presents as a risk to own health and safety.
  - Or the individual presents as a risk to others.

1983 Mental Health Act II

1. I. Section 135 allows the police or other authorised body to enter a private residence and remove a person to a place of safety. An approved social worker must apply to a magistrate's court for a warrant to enable police to enter the premises. The patient can then be taken to an appropriate mental health facility, or police station, for a Mental Health Act assessment. The section lasts up to 72 hours.

2. B. Section 3 is used to detain a patient with a known mental illness for the purpose of administering treatment. This requires an application for detention by the nearest relative or approved social worker and two medical recommendations, one of which must be from a Section 12 approved doctor. The duration of the section is 6 months but after 3 months the patient must give his or her consent to treatment or must be assessed by a second opinion doctor in order for treatment to continue.

3. G. Following sentencing in court, a patient with a mental disorder can be transferred to hospital for compulsory treatment under Section 37 of the Mental Health Act. This may be accompanied by Section 41, which is a restriction order and ensures that the patient is only discharged with the permission of the Home Office.

4. **F.** Patients who are detained in hospital under a section may be granted temporary periods of leave from hospital under Section 17 with permission from the responsible medical officer.

5. **D.** Section 5(2) enables a doctor to hold an inpatient in hospital for up to 72 hours until the patient is formally assessed for a Section 2 or 3. It does not require application by the approved social worker.

Notes

- For patients who are detained under Section 2 or 3, they may appeal against their detention through the Mental Health Review Tribunal or a Hospital Managers' Hearing.

- The table below shows the main mental health regulations used in Scotland and Northern Ireland. Refer to local national legislations for further details.

	Scotland	Northern Ireland
	Part 6	**Article 4**
Admission for Assessment/ short-term detention	• Recommendation by an Approved Medical Practitioner (AMP) and Mental Health Officer (MHO) • Lasts 28 days	• Application made by nearest relative or approved social worker • Recommendation by responsible medical officer on admission • Lasts for seven days and extended by another week
	Part 7	**Article 12**
Detention for treatment	• Application made to Mental Health Review tribunal by MHO • Two medical recommendations required and a care plan • Lasts 6 months • Renewed after 6 months, then every year	• One recommendation from appointed doctor • Lasts for 6 months • Renewed after 6 months, then every year

Ethical issues in psychiatry

1. **A.** The patient's capacity to refuse treatment should be assessed as the surgical team have not assessed her reasons for refusal in their interview. Capacity is not an 'all or nothing' phenomena in that an individual may have the capacity to consent to one procedure but not have the capacity to consent to another. An assessment of capacity requires that the patient *understands* the nature of the proposed treatment, the benefits and risks of the procedure, the risks of not having the procedure, and the nature of any alternative courses of action. The patient must be able to *retain* the information, *arrive* at a decision based on the information given, and to *communicate* this decision. The 2005 Mental Capacity Act of England and Wales states that an individual is considered to have capacity unless proven otherwise.

2. **H.** In this scenario, the patient's delusional thoughts are interfering with his capacity. In emergency situations, patients who lack capacity to consent may be treated in their 'best interests' under the Mental Capacity Act 2005, in order to institute life saving treatment (this was formerly covered by common law). The Mental Health Act does not permit the treatment of medical conditions, unless it is directly related to a psychiatric condition.

3. **B.** The Gillick competence is a test of capacity. A child below the age of 16 years is considered to have Gillick competence if he or she has sufficient understanding and intelligence to understand the nature of the proposed treatment. It must be assessed individually for each child and for each procedure or treatment. A request from a child below the age of 16 years to keep information confidential from his or her parents should be respected unless there are concerns about the child's safety and risk.

4. **I.** The Mental Health Act permits the use of nasogastric feeding in patients with anorexia nervosa, as it is considered a treatment of anorexia nervosa (i.e. a mental illness).

5. **D.** Where a patient has a condition that makes him or her unfit to drive but refuses to stop driving, the General Medical Council advises that patient confidentiality should be broken and the patient should be reported to the UK Driver and Vehicle Licensing Authority (DVLA). This is for the purpose of protecting the safety of others and the patient.

Notes

- Testamentary capacity is the ability to make a valid will. The individual must understand what a will is, appreciate the nature and extent of their property, know the names of potential claimants, and should not be influenced unduly by delusions or an abnormal mental state.

Professionals in psychiatry

1. **F.** When patients are detained in hospital under the 1983 Mental Health Act (MHA), they can appeal their detention to the Mental Health Review Tribunal (consisting of a lawyer, psychiatrist, and a lay member of the public) or the Hospital Managers. Hospital managers are non-executive directors of the hospital trust, who have a specified role under the Mental Health Act and can discharge patients from certain sections via the Hospital Managers' hearing. The nearest relative of the patient can also apply for discharge from detention, but this can be barred by the patient's consultant doctor (responsible medical officer).

2. **H.** Occupational therapists (OTs) aim to promote patient independence through purposeful activities and therapies, such as rehabilitation of interpersonal skills, neuropsychological deficits, and motor function. Assessments of daily living activities such as cooking and cleaning can be assessed by OTs so that they can advise on the level of support the patient requires with their accommodations.

3. **J.** The responsible medical officer (RMO) is the most senior doctor who is in charge of the overall care of the patient, which in many cases is the consultant psychiatrist. For patients who are detained under the MHA, RMOs can grant detained patients temporary leave from the hospital and also discharge them off the MHA sections.

4. **B.** Care coordinators are the named individuals who overlook and coordinate the patient's overall mental and social care needs, usually through the Care Programme Approach (CPA) framework. The role of care coordinators is undertaken usually by community psychiatric nurses, but other professionals such as OTs and social workers also care coordinate patients.

5. C. Clinical psychologists carry out various psychological treatments (psychotherapy), including cognitive behavioural therapy (CBT), psychodynamic psychotherapy, and behavioural therapies. In this scenario, as the patient's drinking appears to be related to temptations from bars and feelings of inadequacy, the psychologist will probably treat the patient with CBT.

Notes

- Approved social workers are social workers trained specifically in dealing with patients with mental health issues. They are authorised under the MHA to apply to hospitals to detain patients against their will if: (1) the patient suffers from a mental illness of a degree and nature requiring inpatient treatment, and (2) the patient presents a risk to self or others.

- The duty doctor is usually a junior doctor in the hospital that covers the hospital unit out of hours to deal with any emergencies.

- The Mental Health Act Administrator is the named person in a mental health unit who coordinates all paperwork and processes relating to the MHA. This involves organising the tribunal, ensuring all necessary documents are in order, and keeping track of dates when certain MHA section expire for specific patients.

- A registered mental nurse is a specially trained nurse in mental health illnesses. They are authorised to temporarily detain at-risk voluntary patients on the ward in the absence of doctors should they try to discharge themselves. In the 1983 MHA, this is conveyed under Section 5(4) and valid for up to 6 hours.

Psychiatric services

1. I. Primary care refers to health care providers that serve as the primary contact with patients in the community, usually through GP and family doctors. In this scenario, the patient drinks slightly above the recommended alcohol limit occasionally but her social life remains undisrupted. Thus simple advice from her GP is all that is required at this point, although if she does develop problem drinking later, she may need to be referred to a community drug and alcohol team (CDAT) for specialist support, such as detoxification, if indicated.

2. A. Assertive outreach teams (AOT) treat people with severe mental illness who have a history of repeated admissions to hospital, complex needs, and poor engagement with other services. They have a smaller case load compared to community mental health teams and thus can provide a more intensive service to engage with difficult patients who may not engage with services otherwise.

3. **G.** Early intervention service (EIS) is an innovative mental health service aimed at identifying and treating young people with a first episode of psychosis. Great emphasis is placed on psychoeducation to teach patients about their illness in order to prevent future relapses and exacerbations. The team also aims to work closely with educational and employment establishments to aid patient re-integration and social recovery.

4. **D.** Community mental health teams (CMHTs) are the main providers of secondary psychiatric care in the community. The team is multidisciplinary but usually headed by a named psychiatric consultant. Patients are managed through outpatient clinics, day visits, and drop-in centres and those requiring further input are allocated a named care coordinator who overlooks the mental and social care needs of patients. CMHT input is indicated in the majority of patients who are discharged from hospital in order to provide continued care in the community.

5. **E.** Crisis resolution teams (CRTs) were created to reduce hospital admissions in patients with severe enduring mental illness presenting in a crisis. They act as gatekeepers to hospital beds and are contacted if an admission to hospital is being considered. They provide a time-limited intervention (medications, psychological, and social input) in the community during the period of crisis. In this scenario, as the patient appears to be in a depressive crisis, time-limited CRT involvement would be best indicated to prevent hospital admission and promote safe recovery at home.

Notes
- Day hospitals are useful for patients who require ongoing monitoring of their mental state but are not acutely unwell to require a hospital admission. They provide structured day activities, including psychotherapy, art therapy, and music groups. Patients often have an individual key worker who will see them on a weekly basis.

- Forensic services are in charge of psychiatric patients involved in the legal systems, and provide inpatient care to such patients in secure units. When indicated, they also provide court reports and legal briefs to provide psychiatric opinions when a psychiatric patient is in court.

- Social services are open to all members of public and provide services for social problems such as housing and child protection. Service is provided by social workers.

CHAPTER 7

Determinants of psychiatric illnesses

Epidemiology of psychiatric illnesses

A. Up to 0.5%
B. 1%
C. 4%
D. 10–20%
E. 25%
F. 28–35%
G. 38%
H. 46%
I. 70%
J. 92%

Select the most appropriate item from the above for each of the following statements.

1. The lifetime risk of schizophrenia in the general population.

2. The risk of schizophrenia in the identical twin of the affected individual.

3. The lifetime risk of unipolar depression in the general population.

4. The incidence of anorexia nervosa in young females.

5. The risk of bipolar affective disorder in the identical twin of the affected individual.

Biological factors of mental illnesses

A. Deficiency of thiamine
B. Deficiency of vitamin B12
C. Deranged melatonin levels
D. Flattening of neuronal discharges on EEG
E. Having an extra chromosome 21
F. Presence of amyloid plaques and neurofibrillary tangles
G. Presence of eosinophilic intracytoplasmic neuronal inclusions with abnormal phosphorylation
H. Raised dopamine sensitivity in neuronal pathways
I. Raised growth hormone level with disruption of the hypothalamic–pituitary–adrenal (HPA) axis
J. Reduced level of serotonin and noradrenaline function in neuronal pathways

Select the most appropriate item from the above that is most likely to be seen in the following scenarios.

1. A 78-year-old male presents with increasing forgetfulness and memory problems. He is unable to look after himself, and his wife has noticed that he has been wandering in the streets at night.

2. A 45-year-old male with a long-standing history of alcohol abuse presents with acute onset confusion and ataxic gait. On examination, he has ophthalmoplegia and nystagmus.

3. A 30-year-old male with several psychiatric admissions in the past presents to hospital complaining that the government is sending signals to his brain to control his thoughts and behaviours.

4. A 25-year-old female presents to the clinic with a 6-month history of low mood, decreased energy, and anhedonia. She is feeling suicidal and has been experiencing insomnia.

5. A 19-year-old female with a BMI of 16 feels that she is overweight. She has not had her menstruation for 4 months.

Risk factors of psychiatric illnesses

A. Associated with female gender, lower social class, and impulsive personality traits.

B. Equal sex distribution in children, but after adolescence, females affected twice as much as males.

C. First-degree relatives are seven times more likely to suffer the same condition.

D. Increased coincidence with mitral valve prolapse.

E. Increased risk associated with obstetric complications and urban births.

F. Predominantly affects females by a male to female ratio of 1:50.

G. Protective factors include smoking and high premorbid intelligence.

H. Risk factors include male gender, being divorced, and having a chronic illness.

I. Schism and skewed parental roles aetiologically implicated.

J. Underlying perfectionist traits and enmeshed family dynamics aetiologically implicated.

For each of the following clinical conditions, select the single most appropriate epidemiological description from the above.

1. Completed suicide

2. Anorexia nervosa

3. Non-fatal deliberate self-harm

4. Depression

5. Schizophrenia

Natural course of psychiatric illnesses

A. Anorexia nervosa
B. Alcohol dependence
C. Alzheimer's disease
D. Bipolar affective disorder
E. Borderline personality disorder
F. Depression
G. Generalised anxiety disorder
H. Obsessive compulsive disorder
I. Puerperal psychosis
J. Schizophrenia

Select the most appropriate diagnosis from the above that best fits with the natural course and prognosis described in each of the following statements.

1. Untreated single episodes of this illness last between 4 and 30 weeks in mild to moderate cases. The risk of subsequent recurrence of similar episodes is roughly 30% at 10 years, rising to over 50% at 20 years.

2. This illness is associated with a prognosis of 20% full recovery, 20% severely ill, and the remainder showing chronic fluctuations. If left untreated, the mortality rate is roughly 10–15%. Poorer prognosis associated with late age of onset and male gender.

3. Long-term prognosis follows the pattern of 1/3 full recovery, 1/3 some improvement, and 1/3 remaining ill, although only roughly 10–20% of those with a first episode will never relapse. Death from suicide is increased 10-fold with this illness.

4. Following an initial episode, the risk of a subsequent disturbance is 90% (40–50% in the first 2 years). Each episode is roughly 6 months long. In a 25-year period, patients may experience roughly 10 episodes.

5. Around two-thirds of cases show improvement by the end of a year, although 20–40% have a chronic course. Poor prognostic factors are early onset, history of personality disorders, and persistent life stressors, while better prognosis is predicted by good premorbid social adjustment and episodic symptoms.

Answers

Epidemiology of psychiatric illnesses

1. **B.** The lifetime risk of schizophrenia in the general population is estimated to be roughly 1%, although some textbooks may quote figures in the range from 0.5% to 1%. With increasing genetic loading, this risk is gradually increased.
   - Schizophrenia affects both males and females equally, but the peak age of onset is younger for males (late teens/early 20s) than females (late 20s).

2. **H.** The risk of schizophrenia in the identical twin of an affected individual is 46%. This highlights the importance of environmental factors as identical twins by definition share all genes. Other useful risk statistics for schizophrenia are:
   - One second-degree relative (e.g. one grandparent): 6%.
   - One first-degree relative (e.g. one parent) affected: 12–15%.
   - Both parents affected: 40%.

3. **D.** The lifetime risk of unipolar depression in the general population ranges between 10% and 20%, but the actual figure is very much dependent on the population surveyed.

4. **A.** The incidence of anorexia nervosa in young females is up to 0.5%, with the peak age of onset being 16–17 years old.

5. **I.** The risk of bipolar affective disorder in the general population is roughly 0.3–1.5%, but if all genetic makeup is shared (as in identical twins), the risk increases to 70%, highlighting the highly heritable nature of the disease.

Notes
- Some environmental factors implicated in schizophrenia are:
  - Maternal viral infections.
  - Winter births (increased incidence in winter births).
  - Complications during pregnancy and birth.
  - Delayed milestones.
  - Urban births.

- The following is a general overview of sex distribution of psychiatric disorders:
  - *More females*: Depressive disorders; anxiety disorders; neuroses in general (including eating disorders and borderline personality disorder); deliberate self-harm; Alzheimer's dementia.

– *More males*: Vascular dementia; suicide; behavioural disruption (dissocial personality disorder, attention-deficit hyperactivity disorder, autism).

– *Equal distribution*: Schizophrenia; bipolar affective disorder; Obsessive-compulsive disorder.

Biological factors of mental illnesses

1. **F.** The diagnosis here is Alzheimer's disease, which is characterised by the presence of amyloid plaques, neurofibrillary tangles, neuronal degeneration, and granulovacuolar degeneration. Cortical acetylcholine is also decreased.

2. **A.** The diagnosis here is Wernicke's encephalopathy resulting from thiamine deficiency as a result of continued alcohol abuse. There are degenerative changes in the thalamus, hypothalamus, and mammillary bodies. Treatment with thiamine reverses the symptoms, but if left untreated, leads to Korsakoff's psychosis, which is irreversible.

3. **H.** The diagnosis here is schizophrenia, and the dopamine hypothesis remains the most accepted theory for the aetiology of psychotic disorders. Evidence for dopamine hyperactivity is demonstrated by the fact that all antipsychotic agents are dopamine D2 antagonists and from the fact that illicit drugs such as amphetamines and cocaine, which are dopaminergic drugs, can cause psychotic symptoms.

4. **J.** The diagnosis here is depression, and the monoamine theory suggests that reduced monoamines such as serotonin and noradrenaline cause depression. Evidence is demonstrated by the fact that antidepressants work by increasing the levels of these monoamines in the brain, and tryptophan (a precursor of serotonin) depletion results in a rapid relapse of depressive symptoms.

5. **I.** The diagnosis here is anorexia nervosa, and raised growth hormone level and disruption of HPA axis are common features. Other endocrine abnormalities include reduced gonadotrophins, raised amylase and cortisol, and reduced T3 thyroid hormones.

Notes

- Deranged melatonin levels are found in seasonal affective disorder.

- Flattening of the EEG may occur in Huntington's disease.

- Lewy bodies are eosinophilic inclusion bodies seen in Lewy body dementia and Parkinson's disease.

- The presence of an extra chromosome 21 is the underlying pathology for Down's syndrome (trisomy 21).

Risk factors of psychiatric illnesses

1. **H:** National rates for suicide vary internationally, but the highest rates are reported in the former Soviet republics of Lithuania, Russia, and Belarus. In the UK, suicide rate is roughly 1/10,000 and accounts for 1% of all deaths. The most common methods are hanging in males and overdoses in females. Associated risk factors are:
   - Three times more common in males.
   - Highest among those aged over 40 years (including the elderly).
   - Social isolation, including divorce/widow, living alone, and unemployment.
   - Psychiatric illnesses associated are depression, alcohol/ substance misuse, schizophrenia, and personality disorders.
   - Previous suicide attempt is the strongest predictor.

2. **J:** Anorexia nervosa affects females 10 times more than males, with a peak incidence at around 16–17 years old. Psychosocial factors are thought to be aetiologically important, and these include enmeshed family dynamics, overprotectiveness, high intra-family conflict, and disturbed body image (self-inflicted, social pressure). Anankastic (obsessive) and perfectionist personality traits are also implicated.

3. **A:** Deliberate self-harm (DSH) accounts for roughly 5–15% of all presentations to general hospitals in the UK, of which 90% are drug overdose. The current estimate in the UK is roughly 3/1000, and the intent behind such acts include a 'cry for help',

desire to get out of an entrapped situation, show desperation to
others, and a true wish to die. Associated risk factors are:
- Rates are higher in female, usually under the age of 35 years.
- Social deprivation, including low social class and unemployment.
- Psychiatric illnesses associated are depression, impulsive personality disorders (dissocial and borderline commonly seen),
and alcohol/substance abuse.
- Previous attempts.

4. **B:** Depression affects both male and female equally until adolescence, but thereafter, female are affected more. The overall
male to female ratio is 1:2.

5. **E:** Schizophrenia certainly has a genetic loading, as incidence is
increased in those with a positive family history. Other associated risks are obstetric and neonatal complications, neurodevel-
opmental delay, maternal influenza in pregnancy, urban setting
at birth, and winter births.
- High expressed emotion in the family is a recognised factor
for *relapse* but not aetiologically implicated. Schism (parental hostility) and skewed parental relationships are no longer
aetiologically implicated although once thought so.

Notes
- Bulimia nervosa affects females 50 times more than males.

- Panic disorder and agoraphobia are associated with increased
rates of mitral valve prolapse, although the aetiological links
between them have not been fully explained.

- Smoking and premorbid intelligence are thought to be protective
factors for Alzheimer's disease.

Natural course of psychiatric illnesses
1. **F.** Depressive episodes are usually self-limiting but the length of
each episode may vary from 4 weeks to 30 weeks, going up to 6
months in severe cases. Subsequent episodes usually require less
stressful events to recur. In severe depressive illness, the suicide
rate may be around 13%, which is 20 times higher compared to
the general population. Poor prognostic factors are comorbid illnesses, insidious onset, neuroticism, and lack of social support.

2. **A.** Anorexia nervosa carries one of the highest mortality rates (10–15%) among psychiatric illnesses, thus signifying the importance of early detection and treatment. Mortality results from physical complications (mainly cardiac) but also due to suicide. Other poor prognostic factors include severe weight loss, chronic illness, and bulimic features.

3. **J.** Schizophrenia is generally associated with poor outcome, with the majority following a relapsing–remitting or severe chronic course. Although half of the patients show some good social functioning, very few remain in paid employment. Poor prognostic factors are insidious onset, negative symptoms, younger age of onset, and long episodes.

4. **D.** Bipolar affective disorder carries a poor prognosis, and after an initial manic episode, up to 90% of patients will have another mood disturbance. With increasing age, the disease-free period between episodes becomes progressively shorter. Poor prognostic factors are psychotic features, depressive features, and treatment non-compliance.

5. **H.** Obsessive-compulsive disorder follows a fairly chronic course with fluctuations in severity of symptoms through life. Poor prognosis is additionally predicted with bizarre compulsions, giving in to compulsions, and comorbid depression.

Notes

- Alcohol misuse and dependency are associated with an increased mortality rate (roughly 3.6 times) compared to age matched controls. Good prognosis is predicted by motivation to change, engagement with treatment, and having a supportive social network.

- Generalised anxiety disorder has a lifetime prevalence of roughly 3–4% and affects females more than males. It has a chronic course with a poor prognosis, exacerbated with substance misuse.

CHAPTER 8
Integrated diagnosis

The psychotic patient

A. Acute and transient psychotic disorder
B. Alcoholic hallucinosis
C. Alzheimer's disease
D. Bipolar affective disorder
E. Delirium
F. Depression with psychotic features
G. Organic delusional disorder
H. Paranoid schizophrenia
I. Schizoaffective disorder
J. Severe obsessive-compulsive disorder with psychotic features

Select the most likely diagnosis from the above for each of the following statements.

1. A 52-year-old female is admitted to a medical ward with an acute exacerbation of Crohn's disease, requiring high-dose steroids and intensive emergency treatment. After a few days, however, she accuses the nurses on the ward of stealing her money and believes that one of the male nurses assaulted her during the night. However, once her steroids are stopped, she starts to settle and no longer voices any bizarre ideations.

2. A 68-year-old male is admitted under the medical team for dehydration after refusing to eat or drink. His wife reports that he has been preoccupied with the belief that he has a brain tumour and has lost pleasure in everything. He has lost 12 kg in weight and spends most of his day in bed. He reports that he can smell rotting bodies and believes that he has committed a sinful crime because he has heard voices calling him a paedophile. He feels ashamed of himself.

3. A 55-year-old female has been writing frequent letters to social services about her neighbours, claiming that they have been plotting to get rid of her. She believes that they are contaminating her water supply with rat poison and as a result has been drinking bottled water only. She has also been cleaning her room meticulously to 'decontaminate' her room. Her daughter says that this has been going on for several months.

4. A 24-year-old male was brought to hospital by the police after being found screaming in the streets. He had apparently followed an elderly couple to their home on many occasions and banged on their door claiming that a divine being was controlling him. On questioning, the patient was very excitable with an incongruous affect. He talked continuously and loudly with marked derailment. He was laughing unstoppably, and claimed that a device in his neck was controlling him and his emotions. His family have been concerned about his whereabouts and state that he had been deteriorating over a period of a few months.

5. A 66-year-old female has been behaving strangely for the last 3 months, accusing her son and daughter-in-law of stealing her belongings. She frequently confuses her 5-year-old grandson with her own son, and believes that her son has been replaced by an imposter. The son reports that she now needs more support with her daily life, as she has stopped looking after herself and has lost weight considerably.

The wandering patient

A. Acute and transient psychotic disorder
B. Alcoholic dementia
C. Alzheimer's disease
D. Delirium
E. Dissociative amnesia
F. Dissociative fugue
G. Korsakoff's psychosis
H. Lewy body dementia
I. Mild cognitive disorder
J. Parkinsons disease

Select the most likely diagnosis from the above for each of the following statements.

1. A 65-year-old female is brought to hospital by the police after she is found wandering the streets in the middle of the night. She cannot recall her address and is disorientated to time and place but not to person. Her consciousness appears intact. Physical examination and blood tests are normal. Her past medical history is unremarkable.

2. A 60-year-old female is brought to hospital after she is found wandering the streets in a town far from her normal residence. Her family reported her missing a few days ago. She appears well kempt but has no recollections of the recent journey that she undertook and her memory for recent events is impaired. Her current memory is fully intact and no signs of cognitive deficits or psychosis are noted. The only significant finding on history is the death of her son 2 weeks ago.

3. A 68-year-old male is brought to hospital after he is found wandering the streets at night. He is disorientated to time, place, and person with a fluctuating level of consciousness. He is agitated and pulls out a cannula that was inserted by a nurse. His behaviour worsens in the middle of the night and he appears to be responding to hallucinations. However, in the morning he is more settled. His urine dipstick suggests that he has a urinary tract infection.

4. A 78-year-old female is brought to hospital after she is found wandering the streets at night. She is disorientated to time, place,

and person. She reports to the nursing staff that she can see children running around the ward. On physical examination she has cogwheel rigidity and a tremor affecting her hands. Her blood tests are normal. Her past medical history is unremarkable.

5. A 50-year-old male is brought to hospital after he is found wandering the streets at night. Consciousness is not impaired but he is disorientated to time and place. Bedside tests reveal that he has a normal digit span and there is no impairment in language and comprehension. When the doctor returns a few hours later the patient is unable to recall their previous meeting and reports that the reason why he is in hospital is because he is visiting a friend. His notes indicate a previous history of excessive alcohol use but he denies current use.

The emotionally labile patient

A. Alcohol intoxication
B. Cocaine intoxication
C. Cyclothymia
D. Emotionally unstable personality disorder
E. Frontal lobe dementia
F. Manic episode
G. Neurosyphilis
H. Pseudobulbar palsy
I. Schizoaffective disorder
J. Vascular dementia

Select the most likely diagnosis from the above for each of the following statements.

1. A 32-year-old female presents to the hospital Emergency Department tearful and screaming after cutting her wrist. Her boyfriend has left her following an intense relationship marked by frequent arguments and physical abuse. She reports a rapidly fluctuating mood and chronic feelings of emptiness.

2. A 28-year-old male is compulsorily admitted to a psychiatric ward. He claims to be a member of the royal family and has been spending money on expensive jewellery and prostitutes, accruing huge debt. On the ward he presents with over-familiarity with the nurses, irritable mood, and labile affect fluctuating from elation to tearfulness within minutes. He also has marked pressure of speech. Physical examination and investigations are normal.

3. A 49-year-old man presents to the hospital Emergency Department in a disinhibited manner. He tries to kiss a female nurse but is held down by the security staff. Following this, he starts screaming and shouting on how badly he is being treated, but he soon becomes tearful and becomes apologetic. He is observed to be unsteady on his feet and his speech is slurred, but he soon falls asleep in the cubicle while waiting for the doctor.

4. The wife of a 50-year-old male complains that her husband has become tactless in his behaviour and she is embarrassed by the sexual gestures he makes towards younger women on the

street. She describes his presentation as 'bubbly' but also being very child like, such as mimicking her actions and speech all the time. He no longer takes care of himself and eats junk food all day. He appears disinterested about everything and believes that his wife is over-reacting. His blood and urine tests are all normal, and his past medical history is unremarkable.

5. A 51-year-old male is admitted to a general medical ward following a cerebrovascular accident. At times he has been observed to be crying and other times he is seen laughing in his room alone. The nurses notice that his speech has become nasal 'like a duck' and that his tongue is stiff and spastic. On examination, his mini-mental state examination score is 27/30.

The restless patient

A. Acute stress reaction
B. Agoraphobia
C. Akathisia
D. Anxious personality disorder
E. Benzodiazepine withdrawal
F. Cannabis intoxication
G. Cocaine intoxication
H. Generalised anxiety disorder
I. Manic episode
J. Social phobia

Select the most likely diagnosis from the above for each of the following statements.

1. An 18-year-old male college student presents to the hospital Emergency Department following a panic attack. He is agitated and is suspicious of nursing staff, claiming that 'they' are against him. On examination, he is tachycardic and has red eyes. There have been no recent stressful events in his life.

2. A 22-year-old male is admitted to hospital for a psychotic illness and was commenced on an antipsychotic medication. Few days later on the ward, he complains of feeling anxious and restless. He is unable to keep his legs from moving and has been pacing up and down the corridors. He is distressed by his symptoms and has been expressing suicidal thoughts. His urine drug screen was negative.

3. A 37-year-old male is brought to hospital by his wife as he has become increasingly irritable and restless over the last 2 weeks. The wife has noticed that he had not been sleeping well and instead is up all night planning business ventures. She also noticed him writing letters to celebrities, claiming that they are his friends. On examination, the patient is highly aroused with marked pressure of speech and flight of ideas.

4. A 19-year-old female student is brought to hospital by her family as she was found heavily hyperventilating and looking 'on the edge'. The patient mentions that on her way home on the

train, she suddenly felt 'suffocated', unsafe, and nervous. She called her family for help and was picked up at the train station, where she was found in a highly agitated and aroused state. Since the attack she has been unable to travel alone by herself and refuses to go back on a train due to her fear of another attack.

5. A 55-year-old female complains of disturbed sleep, weakness, and anxiety. She claims that she can hear high-pitched noises in her ears and also feels as if the world is spinning around. She appears agitated and there is a tremor of her hands. On examination, she is tachycardic. As she is significantly agitated, a full history was not available but she does mention that she recently stopped taking a tablet.

The isolating patient

A. Agoraphobia
B. Anxious personality disorder
C. Depression
D. Normal bereavement reaction
E. Paranoid schizophrenia
F. Paranoid personality disorder
G. Schizoaffective disorder
H. Schizoid personality disorder
I. Schizotypal disorder
J. Social phobia

The following patients display a tendency for solidarity. Select the most likely diagnosis from the above for each of the following statements.

1. A 29-year-old male spends long periods at home doing nothing but surfing on the Internet and solving puzzles. He is currently unemployed, has no real friends, and lives off his parents' income. He has no desire to step out of the house, and only leaves home once a week when he needs to buy cigarettes. When his parents angrily confront him to get a job, he returns to his room to continue with his puzzles.

2. A 40-year-old male has become increasingly socially withdrawn. He believes that the government is monitoring him through a satellite dish because he knows about their plans to poison the head of the monarch. He also believes that they have been trying to remove his thoughts so that no one will find out about their plans. Within the same period he becomes low in mood with decreased energy, anhedonia, and marked psychomotor retardation.

3. A 19-year-old female student becomes anxious when she discovers that she will have to do a presentation in front of her class. She usually has no problems talking to her best friend, but does not speak in class and avoids going to parties for the fear of embarrassing herself in front of others. On the day of the presentation, she starts shaking and blushing, which culminates in a panic attack. She stops attending classes from the following day.

4. A 22-year-old male attended the football team try out and was selected on to the team. When he met his team mates, however, he felt that he was not good enough or cool like the rest of them. He felt very uncomfortable during football practice as he was scared of making mistakes and being told off by others. After a few sessions, he decided not to continue and told everyone that he did not want to injure his ankles or sustain fractures.

5. A 36-year-old female who lost a 10-year-old son a month ago has not been able to leave her house as she finds that she goes through periods where she cannot function normaly with intense tearfulness. She misses her dead son, and has been meticulously cleaning his room everyday after his death as she feels this calms her. When she is not cleaning, she feels increasingly guilty about his death as she starts thinking what she could have done to prevent his death. On some occasions, she claims she can hear him telling her to move on with her life.

The patient that self-harms

A. Anorexia nervosa
B. Bipolar affective disorder
C. Borderline personality disorder
D. Cocaine misuse
E. Depression
F. Dissocial personality disorder
G. Generalised anxiety disorder
H. Lysergic acid diethylamide (LSD) intoxication
I. Malingering
J. Paranoid schizophrenia

The following patients present with evidence of deliberate self-harm. Select the most appropriate item from the above that is the most likely underlying diagnosis in the following scenarios.

1. A 23-year-old male was found cutting his arms and thighs with a knife. He claims that there are bugs crawling underneath his skin and that he is trying to get rid of them. On examination, he is tachycardic with prominent dilatation of pupils and nasal ulceration. He appears sexually disinhibited, restless, and excited.

2. A 20-year-old female presents to hospital having lacerated her forearm. She claims that she had a major argument with her boyfriend and did it so that her boyfriend would worry and not break up with her. According to her, all her relationships in the past have been 'intense like this'. On examination, there are multiple healed laceration scars on both arms.

3. A 65-year-old male was admitted to hospital having stabbed himself in the chest with a knife. On recovery from his wound, he informs the doctor that he did it because he was 'fed up with life' and wanted to die. His wife apparently had died about a year ago and he himself has been suffering from hepatitis and testicular cancer. He feels that there is no future for him.

4. A 38-year-old male presents to hospital with a superficial laceration on his forearm, claiming that he did this as voices were telling him to do it. However, he is unable to describe the exact nature of these voices and his history changes through

the interview. He is insistent on being admitted and wanting a medical certificate excusing him from appearing at court the following day.

5. A 33-year-old male is brought to hospital because he was found cutting his thigh with a knife. He claims that he is a gifted scientist and is under constant surveillance from various intelligence organisations. He apparently has a monitoring chip embedded in his thigh and was using a knife to get rid of it.

Answers

The psychotic patient

1. **G.** This is an example of an organic delusional disorder triggered by an exacerbation of Crohn's disease (linked to psychotic episodes) and use of high-dose steroids (known to trigger manic episodes even in previously well patients). It is not delirium as her consciousness is intact with no suggestions of fluctuating symptoms. A diagnosis of an acute and transient psychotic disorder is also ruled out due to the presence of an organic aetiology.

2. **F.** Depression in older patients may not present with low mood. Mood congruent delusions such as delusions of guilt, poverty, nihilism, and hypochondriasis occur in depression. Olfactory hallucinations of foul odour and second-person auditory hallucinations that are derogatory in nature may also occur. The lack of first-rank symptoms distinguishes this from schizophrenia and schizoaffective disorder.

3. **H.** The most likely diagnosis here is paranoid schizophrenia. Although the patient does present with compulsive cleaning, this is secondary to her delusions. Note that obsessive-compulsive disorder is a neurotic disorder and therefore cannot present with psychotic features such as delusions and hallucinations.

4. **I.** The patient most likely has schizoaffective disorder, since he has moderate symptoms of mania (uninterruptible speech, excitability) coexisting with psychotic features such as delusions of passivity (divine power controlling him, device controlling emotion) and thought disorder. Bipolar affective disorder is a possibility, but the equal presence of affective and psychotic symptoms (including first-rank symptoms) are suggestive of schizoaffective disorder. The longer-time frame also rules out an acute and transient psychotic disorder, which is a schizophrenia-like illness but with duration of less than 4 weeks.

5. **C.** Alzheimer's disease is the most likely diagnosis here, as the patient appears to have experienced a gradual deterioration in function over a period of a few months. She also has memory impairment and is now unable to recall her own grandson. Psychotic symptoms are also common in dementia, particularly persecutory delusions resulting from the patient's deteriorating memory.

Notes

- The hierarchy of diagnosis in psychiatry follows the pattern of: *organic >> psychotic >> affective >> neurotic >> personality disorder.*

The wandering patient

1. **C.** Alzheimer's dementia is the most likely diagnosis as she appears to have memory impairment, consciousness is not impaired, and other causes have been excluded. However, it is important to obtain a collateral history and brain imaging may help to confirm the diagnosis. The main differential is that of delirium, which is marked with fluctuating consciousness.

2. **F.** Dissociative fugue is the most likely diagnosis due to the presence of a recent traumatic event, a purposeful journey away from home, and amnesia for the event. The differential is dissociative amnesia (one of the criteria for dissociative fugue), which is characterised by partial or complete amnesia for recent traumatic events, but no purposeful journey is seen.

3. **D.** Delirium is the most likely diagnosis due to impaired consciousness, psychomotor disturbances, disrupted sleep–wake cycle, fluctuating symptoms, and an underlying organic cause. The main differential diagnoses are dementia and an acute and transient psychotic disorder (an acute onset of delusions and/or hallucinations but consciousness is not impaired and there are no underlying organic causes).

4. **H.** Lewy body dementia is the most likely diagnosis. It is characterised by episodes of confusion, fluctuating cognitive states, visual hallucinations, and parkinsonian features. The main differential is Parkinson's disease, which may present with features of dementia in advanced stages but the patient would normally be diagnosed with Parkinson's disease before then.

5. **G.** Korsakoff psychosis is the most likely diagnosis, characterised by impaired ability to form new memories and a degree of retrograde amnesia. Other aspects of cognition (immediate recall and procedural memory) are normal and patients frequently confabulate to conceal their memory deficits. The main

differential is alcoholic dementia and Alzheimer's dementia, where the abnormalities in cognition are more global.

The emotionally labile patient

1. **D.** Emotionally unstable personality disorder is characterised by instability of mood, with the borderline type further showing chronic emptiness, repeated self-harm, intense relationships, and fear of abandonment. The main differential diagnosis from the list is cyclothymia, which can best be seen as long-term mood swings.

2. **F.** The most likely diagnosis is a manic episode, characterised mainly by his grandiose ideations with risky behaviours and labile affect. The main differential diagnoses are cocaine intoxication and neurosyphilis but his medically cleared status rules them out. Schizoaffective disorder is also another possibility but this patient does not exhibit first-rank symptoms that justify this diagnosis.

3. **A.** Alcohol intoxication is the most likely diagnosis here, as evidenced by his unstable gait, slurred speech, disinhibition, and emotional lability. Other possible differential diagnoses include a manic episode (physical features and sleeping would not be normally seen in acute state) and cocaine intoxication (patient would be more grandiose in presentation with physical features of cocaine intoxication).

4. **E.** Frontotemporal dementia characteristically presents with social disinhibition and changes in personality and behaviour. There is early loss of insight and abnormalities of speech (e.g. perseveration). Cognitive impairment occurs later and the EEG is often normal. Pick's disease is a subtype of frontotemporal dementia. Mania may also present with disinhibition and irritability but other features such as decreased need for sleep, grandiosity, pressure of speech, and flight of ideas distinguishes it from frontotemporal dementia.

5. **H.** The most likely diagnosis here is pseudobulbar palsy, which is an upper motor neurone lesion affecting the muscles involved in eating, swallowing, and talking. The tongue is spastic

and speech is characteristically duck like. The jaw jerk is also increased and emotional lability is common. Recognised causes include cerebrovascular accidents and multiple sclerosis. The main differential here is that of vascular dementia, but it usually presents with cognitive deficits which are usually unevenly distributed and stepwise in deterioration.

The restless patient

1. **F.** Cannabis intoxication is the most likely diagnosis given his paranoid ideations and physical signs such as red eyes. The main differential diagnosis is cocaine intoxication, in which patients can present with grandiose ideations and tachycardia.

2. **C.** Akathisia is a common side effect of antipsychotics (especially typicals) and presents with subjective and motor restlessness. Differential diagnoses include generalised anxiety disorder and substance misuse.

3. **I.** The most likely diagnosis is mania given a 2-week history of gradual increase in manic behaviour and formal thought disorders. The main differential diagnosis is cocaine intoxication, which may present with euphoria, increased energy, grandiose beliefs, and psychotic symptoms but the presentation is more likely to be acute (immediately following use) rather than a build up.

4. **B.** Agoraphobia is an anxiety disorder in which episodes of panic and anxiety are triggered by situations which the individual perceives as being 'unsafe' or unescapable. This may include crowded places and enclosed spaces. In this vignette, the episode of panic was triggered by the patient being in a train.

5. **E.** Benzodiazepine withdrawal presents with transient visual hallucinations, tinnitus, and marked anxiety. This diagnosis is further supported by the fact that the patient recently stopped taking a tablet, most likely a benzodiazepine in this case. Alcohol withdrawal can present with similar symptoms but would not have physical findings such as tinnitus and sensory distortions and the history would be suggestive more of prolonged alcohol dependency.

The isolating patient

1. **H.** The most likely diagnosis here is schizoid personality, as the man in this vignette is withdrawing from social contact and expressing a preference for introspection and solitary activity (surfing the Internet, solving puzzles). He appears content with this lifestyle, and expresses no desire to do anything else or meeting anyone, thus ruling out anxious personality disorder.

2. **G.** A diagnosis of schizoaffective disorder is suggested by the presence of both schizophrenic symptoms and mood disturbance that occur simultaneously during the same episode of illness, and meet the criteria for both disorders. The presence of first-rank symptoms makes depression with psychotic features unlikely.

3. **J.** The female in this vignette most likely has social phobia, as evidenced by her fear of social situations requiring her to mingle with others. The presence of blushing and shaking supports the diagnosis. Anxious personality disorder is a possibility, but not the preferred diagnosis here as she is not necessarily worried about rejection or criticism but more likely a fear of putting herself in the centre of attraction.

4. **B.** Anxious personality disorder is the likely diagnosis in this vignette, as the male constantly feels apprehensive and insecure about his abilities. The perceived risk of sustaining an injury is exaggerated and used as an excuse to withdraw from the team, which fits with anxious personality disorder. Social phobia is unlikely, as he appears to have no problem socialising with others.

5. **D.** Despite the quasi-hallucination and constant rumination about her son's death, these are all part of a normal bereavement reaction and their occurrence is explainable in the context she is in.

The patient that self-harms

1. **D.** Formication is an abnormal skin sensation best described as insects crawling underneath or on the skin. It is a recognised phenomenon in substance misuse, commonly amphetamines (especially cocaine) and alcohol withdrawal. The patient in this

vignette is clearly under the influence of cocaine, and harming himself in response to formication.

2. **C.** Borderline personality disorder is characterised by unstable self-image and emotions, intense relationships, splitting (all-good or all-bad thinking), and pervasive feeling of emptiness. Impulsivity is a core feature and thus patients tend to have recurrent acts of deliberate self-harm.

3. **E.** Depressive illness is a major risk factor for suicide, along with male gender, age over 40 years, chronic illnesses, decreased social support, and a set definite plan. The patient in this vignette presents with a serious suicidal attempt in the context of a depressive episode (marked by pessimism) and psychosocial stressors.

4. **I.** Malingering is the conscious production of symptoms for secondary gain. The patient in this vignette has self-harmed with a clear aim of getting out of obtaining a medical certificate (gain).

5. **J.** Self-harm in schizophrenia can be secondary to delusions and hallucinations, and in this vignette the patient is convinced of the presence of an implanted chip and thus has ended up harming himself.

Notes

- Patients with bipolar manic disorder can put themselves at risk, especially in a manic phase when they present with grandiose delusions of being invincible or divine. In such cases, patients may try to prove their invincibility by jumping from heights or stabbing themselves.

- LSD intoxication is associated with perceptual disturbances, but less commonly with formication.

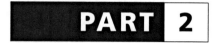

PART 2

Objective structured clinical examinations (OSCEs)

The following are common OSCE stations frequently tested in psychiatry finals for medical students. Each station has a suggested marking scheme covering the basic knowledge and competencies you are required to demonstrate. Remember to modify these schemes according to your examination.

Approaches to objective structured clinical examination stations

Set-up of stations

The objective structured clinical examination (OSCE) consists of several 'stations' which all candidates rotate in turns. Time spent in each station can vary from 5 to 10 minutes depending on the set-up of the station, and within this time, candidates are required to read the instructions and carry out the specified tasks.

Types of station

OSCEs in psychiatry can usually be broken down into three types:
1. *Interview*: Candidates are required to take a history, in particular focusing on the history of presenting complaint to obtain enough details to make a diagnosis. They may also be asked to focus on a particular aspect of the mental state examination (MSE), such as thought processes to elicit specific delusions. The overall aim of these stations is to test whether the candidates can adequately carry out assessments.
2. *Communication*: These stations involve discussing a specific treatment or disorder with the patient or the carer, and great emphasis is placed on explaining medical jargon in simple English.
3. *Practical*: This refers to any station that does not require active conversation with the patient, but rather practical tasks. It may involve patients (such as physical examination) or stand-alone stations.

General tips for psychiatry OSCEs

1. Remember that OSCEs are artificial situations, with simulated patients, simple scenarios, and unrealistic time limits. The very nature of psychiatry makes OSCE a difficult experience because in real life situations, you will not assess a patient in 5 minutes. The aim of OSCEs therefore is to act the role of a doctor (or any role in the instruction) in the given time, and to complete the

189

given task in the allotted time to the best of your ability. You may thus have to speed up in certain parts of the station.

2. Read the instructions and do specifically what it tells you to do. If the instruction is to obtain a history to make a diagnosis of PTSD, do not waste your time going through management as you will not get any marks on it.

3. Each examiner is equipped with a predetermined checklist, and marks your performance as to whether you completed each task or not. You should aim to broadly cover all the possible areas for a given task, because if you do not cover something, you will not get marks for that particular tick box. Your goal is not to shine in one particular area, but to collect as many marks as possible to help you pass.

4. Keep track of time. If you find that you are spending too much time on one specific aspect and are getting nowhere, move on and cover other areas.

Tips for interview-type stations

1. For any station, communication skills are crucial and carry a sizeable proportion of marks. You must be empathic in your approach to the patient and build rapport. You must be seen to be non-judgmental and friendly, as this will help the patient (actor) ease up and facilitate disclosure of information.

2. Use lots of open questions in the initial stages of the interview, such as 'How can I help you today?' or 'Please tell me about …' From there, use narrow questions to clarify certain aspects of the history or mental state.

3. The majority of history and assessment stations are straightforward with very specific instructions on what is required. If the station asks for a diagnosis, the bulk of your interview should focus on obtaining a good history of presenting complaint, covering:
   - Nature of the problem.
   - Onset, duration, and frequency of problem.
   - Precipitating events.
   - Alleviating or exacerbating factors.

4. Think broadly, and remember the bio-psycho-social model of psychiatric illnesses.

5. If you get stuck or decide to ask other aspects of the history, the following mnemonic should be useful: *PRAMS* (*Past* psychiatric history, *Risk* to self and others, *Alcohol* and drug use, *Mood*, *Social* functioning).

Tips for communication-type stations

1. A useful starting point with these stations is to enquire about how much background information the patient or carer already knows, and whether they have any specific concerns they would like to address.
2. Remember to use simple language and avoid medical jargon, including acronyms. You need to be able to explain things in simple English.
3. In psychiatry, many diseases have no known single cause. It is perfectly acceptable to say that the causes are multifactorial and briefly mention some known factors. But remember to be sensible and sensitive.
4. Structure your response so that it is easy to follow and covers all adequate areas. The minimum areas that you would be expected to cover depends on what is being asked.
   - *Disease*: Definition, causes, treatments (bio-psycho-social), prognosis.
   - *Treatment*: Definition, administration, benefits, side effects, monitoring.

Practical stations

Practical stations cover a very wide range, but at the minimum, they can be split into those that are 'medical' or 'psychiatric'.

The emphasis on 'medical' stations depends on the curriculum of each school, but this may include simple physical examinations such as a neurological examination of the limbs or cranial nerves, commenting on CT scans, and interpreting blood results (infections, thyroid diseases, lithium toxicity).

Psychiatric practical stations that may appear in OSCE examinations include:

- Going through the 30-point mini-MSE.
- Written stations on mental health legislation practicalities.
- Written stations on ECT practicalities.
- Written stations on rapid tranquillisation practicalities.

Hints for the MSE

The MSE is a core component of any psychiatric history and allows the psychiatrist to obtain a snap-shot picture of the patient's mental state at a given point in time. In OSCEs, you may be asked to examine parts of the MSE with an actor, or to watch a video and make an overall comment.

Components of a typical MSE are listed below. The majority of these can be obtained through observation or during the interview, but some of them (such as mood, perception, thought content, insight, and cognition) do need to be explored specifically.

Appearance and behavior: What is the patient wearing? Are they appropriate? Any distinguishable features such as tattoos? Is the patient displaying any abnormal movements? Any signs of psychomotor retardation or agitation? How is the patient's eye contact? What is the level of rapport established?

Speech and thought form: What is the rate, tone, and volume of the patient's speech like? Are the sentences constructed meaningfully and does it make sense? Any signs of formal thought disorders such as loosening of association?

Mood and affect: The patient's mood needs to be assessed, such as: 'How have you been feeling recently?' Biological features such as appetite, sleep, and motivation also need to be ascertained. Observe how the patient objectively looks, and comment on whether this matches with what the patient expresses.

Thought content: Is the patient expressing anything that may be out of the ordinary? If so, the intensity with which those thoughts are held need to be explored, for example: 'You mentioned that there were people coming after you. How would you react if someone says that it does not make sense?' Risk issues such as homicidal and suicidal thoughts also need to be clarified.

Abnormal perception: Enquire specifically whether the patient is experiencing abnormal perceptions such as auditory or visual hallucinations. These should be sensibly asked, such as: 'Have you had strange experiences when you were able to hear people talking when there was no one around, or when others around you couldn't hear them?'

Cognition: Ideally this should be tested using the 30-point mini-MSE. If this is not practical, at the minimum, the patient's orientation to time, place, and person needs to be assessed. ('Do you know where you are now? What is the time now? Can you tell me your full name and date of birth?')

Insight: This is the patient's own understanding about his or her condition, and whether they agree that they have a mental illness and agree to receive treatment. ('I see that you are going through a lot at the moment. What do you think is the cause of this? Would you be willing to accept hospital treatment for it?')

The above should be used as a guide so that they can be modified according to the requirements of the individual OSCE stations you might come across.

1
History and assessment: Depression

Scenario: *A 30-year-old female was brought to hospital by her partner as she has not been eating well. Assess this patient with a view to making a diagnosis.*

Notes: Try to establish the core depressive symptoms of depression and its severity using the ICD-10 or DSM-IV criteria. Risk of self-harm, including suicide, needs to be explored.

Checklist of core knowledge

Assessment of mood and its severity
- Low mood for at least 2 weeks.
- Loss of interest or pleasures (anhedonia).
- Decreased energy level.
- Beck's cognitive triad: Loss of confidence? Negative view of world? Hopelessness?
- Any diurnal changes in these thoughts.

Assessment of somatic features
- Difficulty concentrating or thinking.
- Change in psychomotor activity such as agitation or retardation.
- Sleep disturbance, including insomnia and early morning waking.
- Change in appetite, and any corresponding weight changes.
- Reduced sexual energy.

Risk to self
- Any thoughts of death or suicide?
- Any previous attempts.

Extra questions

- Any similar episodes in the past? If so, a diagnosis of recurrent depressive disorder needs to be considered.
- Previous episodes of mania or hypomania to rule out bipolar affective disorder.
- Previous treatments received, including psychiatry outpatient appointments and hospital admissions.
- Any current medications and compliance.
- Use of illicit substances and alcohol, and any recent change in consumption of these.
- Mental state: Presence of delusional thinking? Auditory or visual hallucinations?
- If in the context of childbirth, what is the risk to the newborn baby?

2
History and assessment: Bipolar affective disorder

Scenario: *A 23-year-old female was brought to hospital by her family because of increasing disruptive behaviour. Assess this patient with a view to establishing a diagnosis.*

Notes: Try to establish the core manic symptoms and examine their severity. A hypomanic person often comes across as being energetic and overfamiliar, while a manic person can present as elated and difficult to interview due to marked pressure of speech and distractibility. Risk of harm to self needs to be explored, including vulnerability and exploitation.

Checklist of core knowledge

Core manic symptoms
- *Mood*
  - Elated mood, feeling 'high in spirits'.
  - Signs of irritability.
- *Physical*
  - Increased physical activity and restlessness.
  - Difficulty concentrating.
  - Decreased need of sleep.
  - Increased sexual energy.
- *Stream of thought*
  - Flight of ideas or subjective feeling of racing thoughts.
  - Increased talkativeness.
- *Behavioural*
  - Presence of reckless and impulsive behaviours, such as spending sprees, excessive drinking, and dangerous driving.
  - Presence of disinhibited behaviour that is out of character, for example engaging in intimate activities with strangers.
  - Increased grandiosity and self-esteem.

Circumstances of these symptoms

- How long has this been going on? How frequent are they?
- Any known triggers?
- Disruption to work and social life: severe disruption seen in mania.

Mental state examination: Psychotic features can be seen in mania

- Delusional beliefs, often of grandiose nature (e.g. Special powers, being famous).
- Hallucinations, often auditory (usually second person) or visual.

Risk issues

- Reckless activities which may put self or others at risk.
- Is the patient being exploited by others as a result of increased vulnerability?

Extra questions

- Any previous episodes of mania/hypomania or depression?
- Previous or current medications and treatments, including hospital admissions.
- Any use of drugs prior to onset to manic episode?

3
History and assessment: Anxiety disorders

Scenario: *A 43-year-old female presents to the clinic complaining of feeling 'on the edge' all the time. Take a history with a view to establishing her diagnosis.*

Notes: Establish the core symptoms of anxiety, and try to work out the specific diagnosis. Assess the impact of these symptoms on the patient's life.

Checklist of core knowledge

Anxiety symptoms
- *Physical*: Palpitations, sweating, shakiness, difficulty breathing, chest discomfort, nausea, light-headedness, dizziness, dry mouth, restlessness.
- *Psychological*: Feeling unreal, fear of 'going crazy', fear of losing control over one's self, feeling that death is imminent, inability to relax, nervousness.
- Onset, duration, and frequency of symptoms.

Circumstances of symptoms
- *Generalised anxiety disorder*: Anxiety symptoms present all the time. Worry and tension about everyday things. Symptoms present for at least 6 months, with no real trigger.
- *Panic disorder*: Discrete episodes arising spontaneously and abruptly with no identifiable causes, often resolving in a few minutes.
- *Agoraphobia*: Episodes of anxiety occurring when in crowded places, public places, or any place away from a 'safe' place (commonly home).
- *Social phobia*: Fear of being the focus of attention, or any potential embarrassment.

- *Specific (simple) phobia*: Marked anxiety in response to a specific object, place, situation. Examples include snakes, spiders, blood, and water.

Psychosocial impact of anxiety symptoms
- Avoid any specific situations or objects due to fear of getting an anxiety episode?
- Impact on daily living and social life, such as jobs and friends.
- Any change in use of alcohol and illicit substance, as patients may be self-medicating to relieve their anxiety symptoms.
- Presence of any depressive symptoms.

Extra questions
- Questions on thyroid function (weight loss, heat intolerance, excessive sweating) to rule out hyperthyroidism as a potential cause of anxiety disorders.
- Current medications, to check for any drug interactions causing anxiety and also to rule out any benzodiazepine dependence to cope with anxiety.
- Presence of 'anticipatory anxiety' (anxiety experienced as one constantly anticipates an attack of anxiety).
- Risk assessment: Has the anxiety been so bad to the point that they felt like doing something to themselves?

4

History and assessment: Obsessive-compulsive disorder

Scenario: *A 26-year-old female was referred by her company's occupational health department as she does not appear to be coping at work. Assess this patient with a view to making a diagnosis.*

Notes: Use the ICD-10 criteria as a basis to get a comprehensive history on obsessions and compulsions. The effects of these symptoms on the patient's social life and mental health need to be assessed.

Checklist of core knowledge

Assess the nature and quality of obsessions and compulsions
- These must be present for 2 weeks.
- Obsessions are thoughts, ideas, ruminations, and doubts that enter the patient's mind repeatedly and cause distress.
- Compulsions are non-purposeful acts or rituals (e.g. counting, washing, checking) that are carried out repeatedly. They often follow rules and have a 'magical' quality.

Core features of obsession and compulsions
- Acknowledged as originating in own mind, and not by some alien force.
- Repetitive and unpleasant, and acknowledged as unreasonable.
- Patient tries to resist them, but unsuccessfully to a degree.
- Experience is not pleasurable in itself.

Impact on life
- Causes distress.
- Interferes with patient's social functioning, such as relationships, employment, and interests.

Risk issues
- Enquire about depression and anxiety disorders.
- Any thoughts of harming self.
- Enquire about alcohol and drugs resulting from the strain of these symptoms.

Extra questions
- Rule out psychotic symptoms and any other comorbid illnesses (such as depression and other anxiety disorders).
- Pharmacological treatments: commonly use selective serotonin reuptake inhibitors.
- Psychological treatments: behavioural therapies (such as graded exposure and response prevention), or cognitive behavioural techniques.

5

History and assessment: Eating disorders

Scenario: *A 19-year-old female is brought to hospital by her family as she has lost 10 kg in the last 2 months. Assess the patient with a view to making a diagnosis.*

Notes: Establish current eating patterns, and assess for anorexia and bulimia nervosa. Physical aspects should also be enquired as patients may be putting their lives at risk.

Checklist of core knowledge

Eating pattern
- Frequency and quantity of eating in a typical day.
- How did the eating pattern change over time?
- Current height and weight (to calculate BMI).
- Ideal weight and her lowest and highest recorded weight.

Common features of anorexia and bulimia
- Intrusive fear of fatness and self-perception that they are fat.
- Weight-losing behaviour:
  - Avoidance of 'fattening' food with periods of starvation.
  - Self-induced vomiting or purging.
  - Use of medications such as appetite suppressants, diuretics, and thyroid medications.
  - Excessive exercise.

Specific features of anorexia
- BMI less than 17.5, or weight at least 15% below that expected.
- Disruption of hypothalamus–pituitary axis, manifesting as amenorrhoea in females and loss of sexuality and potency in males.

Specific features of bulimia

- Persistent desire or compulsion to eat (craving).
- Recurrent episodes of binge eating, at least twice a week for 3 months.
  - What does the patient eat during a binge and over what length of time?
  - How does the patient feel after the binge? (self-loathing, feelings of disgust).

Extra questions

- Physical symptoms such as lethargy and muscle weakness as there are high risks of medical complications.
- Comorbid depression and rule out risk of suicide.
- *Premorbid personality*: Patients with anorexia are likely to be anankastic with traits for perfectionism, while bulimia is associated with impulsivity.
- *Family and personal history*: Enmeshment (intense) relationship within family? Family history of eating disorders? Occupation such as models and ballerinas at high risk.
- Offer to conduct a physical examination (dehydration, bradycardia, hypotension, peripheral neuropathy, loss of power, dental carries, thin hair, lanugo hair); ECG (prolonged QT interval, arrhythmia); bloods (hypothyroidism, hypokalaemia, hyponatraemia, low glucose, hypercortisolaemia, anaemia).

6

History and assessment: Post-traumatic stress disorder

Scenario: *A 31-year-old female presents to her doctor for poor sleep and lack of appetite, which had started about a month ago when she was attacked on her way back from work. Take a history with a view to making a diagnosis.*

Notes: Other comorbid psychiatric disorders are common. Make sure depression, other anxiety disorders, and the use of illicit drugs are enquired.

Checklist of core knowledge

Establish a relationship between the incident and symptoms
- Onset of PTSD symptoms should be within 6 months of the traumatic event.
- What are the core symptoms experienced? How frequent are they?

Core symptoms of PTSD
- *Exposure to an exceptionally threatening situation or event*
  - Account of the event, and the patient's emotional response to the incident.
  - Did she sustain any injuries?
- *Persistent remembering or 're-living' of the event*
  - Any recurrent and intrusive memories of the attack?
  - Distressing dreams or nightmares?
  - 'Flashbacks' of the attack?
  - Distress at being exposed to situations associated with the event?

- *Avoidance of events related to the stressor*
  - Does she avoid thinking or talking about the event?
  - Does she avoid activities or places associated with the event? Has she been back to the crime scene?
  - Are there any feelings of detachment or numbness?
- *Difficulty recalling the incident*
  - Does she have any problems remembering an important aspect of the incident?
- *Persistent symptoms of increased arousal*
  - Does she startle easily?
  - Does she have difficulty concentrating?
  - Does she have problems with her sleep?
  - Does she lose her temper easily or become irritable?

Mental state examination
- Current mood, including suicidal ideation?
- Any comorbid psychiatric disorders?

Past history
- Any past psychiatric history?
- What was the patient's premorbid personality like?

Social functioning
- What is the current level of social support?
- How have the symptoms affected her work, family, and social life?
- How has she been coping? Has she been using drugs or alcohol?

7

History and assessment: Psychotic illness

Scenario: *A 17-year-old male was brought to hospital by his family with a 2-month history of increasingly bizarre behaviour and marked social withdrawal. Assess the patient with a view to establishing a diagnosis.*

Notes: Using Schneider's first-rank symptoms or the ICD-10 criteria as a basis, try to establish what psychotic phenomena the patient is experiencing and assess any risks.

Checklist of core knowledge

Major psychotic symptoms: Establish onset and duration, as ICD-10 requires 1-month duration of the following symptoms

- *Delusional beliefs*: Unshakeable, culturally inappropriate, and not plausible
  - Types of delusions include persecutory, grandiose, infidelity, nihilistic, etc.
  - Need to test for strength of these delusional beliefs.
  - Delusional perception: a normal perception that is given a delusional meaning.
- *Auditory hallucinations*: Number of voices; male/female; where do they come from
  - Running commentary.
  - Third-person discussion about the patient.
  - Hearing thoughts spoken out loud (thought echo).
- *Abnormal thought processes*
  - Thought insertion: Any thoughts transmitted into your head that is not yours?
  - Thought broadcast: Thoughts spoken out loud so that others can hear?
  - Thought withdrawal: Are thoughts taken out from your head so that your mind goes blank?

- *Passivity phenomena*
  - Delusional belief that one's actions, feelings, or impulses are controlled externally.
  - Complaints that body parts are being controlled against own will.

Other symptoms
- Persistent hallucinations in other modalities.
- *Disorders of thought formation*: Neologisms (new words), loosening of association (breaks in train of thought), incoherent/irrelevant speech.
- *Abnormal repetitive movements (catatonia)*: Excitement, maintenance of postures for long periods, mutism.
- *Negative symptoms*: Marked apathy, emotional blunting, marked withdrawal, reduced drive.

Risk issues
- How is the patient coping with these psychotic symptoms?
- Is the patient doing anything in response to these symptoms, and putting self and others at risk?

Extra questions
- Any use of illicit substances?
- What is the patient's insight into these symptoms?
- Level of current social functioning, and impact on life.
- Previous psychiatric history.
- Family history.

8

History and assessment: Puerperal psychosis

Scenario: *A 28-year-old female was brought to hospital with her 3-week-old baby. Her parents report that she has been behaving strangely and neglecting the baby. Assess this patient with a view to establishing the diagnosis.*

Notes: Safety and risk to the mother, baby, and others need to be explored. Consider predisposing psychosocial risk factors. The main puerperal disorders are puerperal depression and psychosis. Puerperal psychosis is the most important illness to rule out due to the risk of harm to the baby. Puerperal psychosis may present with affective psychotic symptoms and schizophrenic symptoms.

Checklist of core knowledge

Presenting features of puerperal psychosis
- *Onset:* Puerperal Psychosis usually presents within the first 2 weeks of labour.
- Presents with insomnia, irritability, and restlessness.
- *Features of mania may be present:* Elation, overactivity, pressure of speech, labile mood, grandiosity.
- *There may be depressive symptoms:* Low mood, low energy, anhedonia, negative thoughts.
- *Psychotic symptoms:* Persecutory delusions about the baby (baby is deformed, evil) and of others, delusions of passivity, auditory hallucinations (including command hallucinations of harming the baby).

Presenting features of puerperal depression: to be ruled out
- Puerperal depression presents within the first 6–8 weeks of labour.
- Presents with tearfulness and irritability.

- Feelings of being an inadequate mother.
- Concerns about the baby's health.
- Insomnia, decreased appetite and libido, and poor concentration.

Risk
- Neglect of baby and self.
- Thoughts about harming the baby (including command hallucinations).
- Thoughts about harming self.

Predisposing factors
- Complications during and after pregnancy (e.g. delivery by caesarean section and instrumental delivery) increase risk of puerperal psychosis.
- Lack of support during and after pregnancy increases risk of both disorders.
- First pregnancy associated with increased risk of puerperal psychosis.
- Previous history or family history of bipolar affective disorder or puerperal psychosis increases risk of puerperal psychosis.

Other questions
- Current medication.
- If similar episode occurred in the past – What treatment did she receive? (including ECT).
- Use of illicit substances and alcohol.

9
History and assessment: Alcohol history

Scenario: *A 63-year-old male presented to hospital with a fall. A routine blood test showed deranged liver function tests. He wants help with his alcohol problems. Take an alcohol history and establish the presence of dependency.*

Notes: Establish the drinking pattern of the patient, and then screen for dependence. Associated risks of continued drinking need to be assessed.

Checklist of core knowledge

Alcohol consumption
- Quantify amount of alcohol consumed in a typical day and week in units (one unit is equivalent to a half-pint of beer or a glass of wine).
- *Type of alcohol consumed*: Any type of alcohol, or just one type (stereotyped drinking).
- When does the drinking occur during the day? Is the patient using alcohol from the moment they wake up?
- Who do they drink with (alone or with someone else)?

Establishing dependence (ICD-10)
- Strong desire or sense of compulsion to drink.
- Difficulty controlling the amount drunk.
- Evidence of tolerance, as evidenced by the need to consume larger amounts to get the desired effect.
- Preoccupation with alcohol, leading to progressive neglect of other activities.
- Persistent use despite evidence of harmful consequences.
- Presence of physiological withdrawal symptoms when drinking stops.

Effects of alcohol

- *Acute withdrawal*: Tremor, sweating, nausea, tachycardia, high blood pressure, headache, insomnia, psychomotor agitation.
- *Delirium tremens*: Acute psychotic episode occurring on alcohol withdrawal, often presenting with acute confusion, formication ('insects crawling under skin'), and visual hallucinations (snakes, rats, insects, etc.).
- *Withdrawal fits*: Grand mal seizures resulting from alcohol withdrawal. Can be fatal if left untreated, so presence of previous fits (and any treatment received) must always be asked.
- *Other medical complications*: CNS (Korsakoff's psychosis and Wernicke's encephalopathy), gastrointestinal (peptic ulcers, oesophageal varices), liver (cirrhosis).
- *Psychological complications*: Depression, anxiety, morbid jealousy, alcoholic hallucinosis.

Risk issues

- How do they fund their drinking? Do they engage in crime to fund their addiction?
- Any previous problems with the police?
- Use of illicit substances.

Extra questions

- *Risk factors*: Occupation (journalists, doctors), family history, past psychiatric history.
- Impact on family and social life.

10

History and assessment: Opiate misuse and risk minimisation

Scenario: *A 27-year-old male presents to hospital with a large abscess in his groin. He is referred by the Emergency Department doctor as the patient admitted to using heroin and does not want to give up. Obtain a brief drug history and provide advice to minimise any risks involved.*

Checklist of core knowledge

History of drug use
- Progression of types of drugs used in the past, including duration and periods of abstinence.

Opiate history
- Amount of opiate currently taken.
- Cost of buying the drugs, including methods of funding.
- *Methods of administration*: Smoking, injecting.
- First time opiate used.
- How frequent currently?
- *Brief enquiry about dependence*: Craving, withdrawal symptoms, tolerance.

Motivational interviewing
- What are the good points of using heroin?
- What are the bad points?
- How has heroin affected his life?
  - Any effects on physical or mental health?
  - Any overdoses?
- Have you ever thought of cutting down on your heroin use?
  - If previous attempts to seek abstinence, what happened? What triggered the relapse?

– Any anxiety if trying to cut down?

– What do you think will happen if you try to cut down?

Risk minimisation

- To prevent any possible overdoses, do not take heroin when alone.

- If injecting, appropriate advice needs to be given about using clean needles, and that none of the injection apparatus (needles, syringe, filter, spoon) should be shared. This is to prevent any infection with blood-borne viruses such as HIV and hepatitis.

  – If previous history of sharing needles, advise getting an infection screen.

  – Advise on alternative methods of using heroin, such as smoking.

  – If adamant on injecting, advice patient to rotate injection sites and avoid injecting in neck, groin, or any infected areas.

- Avoid using opiates with any other drugs, as it may interact.

- Discuss about methadone replacement as an alternative to using heroin, or managed detoxification.

  – Methadone is a sugar-less liquid which can be prescribed by specialist substance misuse units, and they are dispensed daily from a pharmacist.

- Enquire about any social problems, and offer to make referrals to appropriate agencies involved, such as housing associations if homeless.

- If the patient is not registered with a doctor, encourage to obtain a primary care doctor.

- Any previous psychiatric history? (Drugs can exacerbate psychiatric symptoms). Is the patient receiving regular review if mental illness present?

11

History and assessment: Risk assessment for suicidality

Scenario: *A 38-year-old male is brought to hospital after taking a serious overdose of paracetamol. Assess the level of risk.*

Notes: It is essential to be sensitive and empathic when assessing a suicidal patient. As well as establishing the facts of what has already happened, assess risk of ongoing suicidal ideation and future acts.

Checklist of core knowledge

Antecedents of the suicidal act
- Events leading to the act, including psychosocial stressors.
- *Degree of preparation for the act*: Any last acts, such as suicidal note or a will?
- Was the act impulsive or planned?

Circumstances of the suicidal act
- What did the act consist of? For example, if an overdose, what was taken? Was the patient under the influence of alcohol or illicit substances?
- Where and when did the act take place? Was the act performed in isolation? Were any precautions taken to prevent being found?

Consequences of the suicidal act
- How did the patient come to medical attention?
- What was the true intention of the act? To really die or 'cry for help'?
- Did the patient believe at the time that the act would be lethal?
- How does the patient feel about the act now?

Current risk
- How does the patient feel about the future?
- Current mood?
- Any further plans to harm self? What is stopping them from carrying out those acts?

Past psychiatric history
- Previous attempts of self-harm or suicide.
- Current or past psychiatric diagnosis, including treatment.

Extra questions
- Mental state examination to assess presence of delusional beliefs and psychotic symptoms.
- Family history of psychiatric illnesses and suicide.
- Social circumstances, such as support network and accommodation issues.
- Use of alcohol and illicit substances.

12

History and assessment: Risk assessment for violence

Scenario: *A 32-year-old male believes that his wife has been having an affair with their next door neighbour. He has become increasingly agitated. Assess this man's risk to others.*

Notes: Risk to be assessed for self, known others, and indiscriminate others. For a given incident, risk assessment involves assessing the precipitants, index incident, and the consequences. This is then compared with the patient's previous history of risk and mental state. Current mental state (for delusions, hallucinations, suicidality, etc.) is then assessed.

Checklist of core knowledge

History of presenting complaint
- Explore his thoughts about the affair – could these thoughts be delusional in nature (morbid jealousy)? What evidence does he have for the affair?
- Does he have any other delusions such as delusions of thought insertion, withdrawal, or broadcast? Delusions of passivity?
- Has he been hearing voices – any command hallucinations asking him to harm others?
- Are there any disturbances in mood such as depression or elated mood?
- Have there been any recent psychosocial stressors?

Risk
- Does he feel angry about the affair? Does he have any plans to confront or attack his partner or her alleged partner?
  - If so, what does he plan to do? What preparations has he made for this?
- Does he have any suicidal ideation?

Past psychiatric history
- Does he have a history of psychosis, depression, or substance misuse?
- Is he currently on medication and has he been compliant?
- Does he have a history with disengagement with services?

Substance misuse
- Does he have a history of alcohol dependence or substance misuse?
- Any substance misuse currently?

Forensic history
- Does he have a history of violence or aggression?
- What were the circumstances surrounding previous acts of violence – Were they impulsive or planned? Did he use a weapon? Did he know his victims?
- Has he been convicted of any crimes?

Personality
- Are there any features of dissocial personality disorder? Tendency to blame others, lack of guilt or remorse for actions, inability to learn from mistakes, low frustration threshold, impulsivity, and a tendency to get into fights.

Social history
- Is he currently homeless?
- Does he have any social support?
- Any other psychosocial stressors, such as financial difficulties?

13

Communication: Schizophrenia

Scenario: *A 23-year-old male was admitted to hospital with a first episode of schizophrenia. His mother would like to see you to discuss his illness, and has his permission to do so. Address her concerns regarding her son's illness.*

Checklist of core knowledge

What is schizophrenia?
- It is a serious mental disorder that affects 1 in every 100 people.
- People with schizophrenia can have problems distinguishing what's real and what's not, and this affects the way they think, feel, and behave. As a result, they can come up with strange ideas (delusions), or hear and see things that aren't really there (hallucinations).
- Contrary to popular belief, schizophrenia is not 'split mind', and people with schizophrenia are rarely dangerous or unpredictable.

What caused it?
- We do not know the exact cause of schizophrenia. Genetic background may partly account, as having a parent with schizophrenia can increase the risk by 10 times. However, other factors such as birth complications and drug use can affect the brain and may play a role.
- Stressful life events do not in themselves cause schizophrenia, but they are important triggers in bringing on the illness in susceptible individuals.

What medications are used in treating schizophrenia?
- Antipsychotics (or neuroleptics) is the main class of medication used in treating schizophrenia. People with schizophrenia often have an imbalance (excess) of a brain chemical called dopamine

during an acute psychotic episode, and antipsychotics aim to correct the balance.

- There are two types of antipsychotics, typical and atypical. Typical antipsychotics (e.g. haloperidol) are older but we have more experience with them and they are good in alleviating disturbing symptoms. Atypical antipsychotics (e.g. olanzapine) are newer and appear to be effective across a wider range of symptoms (positive and negative symptoms).

What are the side effects of using these medications?

- With the older typical antipsychotics, common side effects encountered are stiffness, restlessness (akathisia), sleepiness, blurring of vision, and involuntary movements of facial and neck muscles. They are termed extrapyramidal side effects (EPSEs).
- The newer atypical antipsychotics cause less EPSEs, but instead may cause weight gain, sexual dysfunction, diabetes, hypertension, hypercholesterolaemia, and neutropaenia.

Are there any other treatments?

- Psychological treatments can be used alongside medication and these include family therapy and cognitive behavioural therapy.

What are the future prospects?

- The medications only control the symptoms and do not cure schizophrenia.
- Roughly 20% of people with schizophrenia recover completely after the first episode, but 70% will have breakdowns (acute episodes) in the future. Continuing to take medications will decrease the chances of these breakdowns from happening.
- The community mental health team (CMHTs) consisting of psychiatrists, psychologists, therapists, and nurses can provide your family with the necessary support in the community.

14
Communication: Alzheimer's disease

Scenario: *A 65-year-old male was just told that his wife has a likely diagnosis of Alzheimer's disease. Address any concerns he may have about his wife's diagnosis.*

Checklist of core knowledge

What is Alzheimer's disease?

- With increasing age, everyone loses brain cells and the ability to learn new information becomes harder. In Alzheimer's disease, there are changes in brain structures (amyloid plaques, neurofibrillary tangles, loss of cortical mass) and chemicals (acetylcholine) which make this process more severe and rapid than normal ageing.

How did she get this?

- Alzheimer's disease tends to run in certain families, but this is limited mainly to cases when the disease appears early in life. In the vast majority of people, however, there is no clear set pattern of inheritance.

Will she ever get better?

- Unfortunately the disease is progressive, meaning that symptoms can become worse as more parts of the brain are affected.
- Initially she may just be forgetful or wander, but as the disease becomes severe, there may be problems with practical tasks like cooking, cleaning, and dressing. She may also develop problems with her speech and her ability to recognise objects and people.

Are there treatments available?

- No medication can stop the progression of Alzheimer's disease, but there are medications that we can use in the initial stages that will slow the progression of the illness. They can reduce anxiety, agitation, and the rate of memory loss.

• Commonly used medications are donepezil, rivastigmine, and galantamine (all of them are acetylcholinesterase inhibitors), which try to maintain a steady level of the chemical acetylcholine in the brain. This chemical is important for transmission of information.

• Some of the side effects of these medications are sleep disturbances, nausea, loss of appetite, diarrhea, and muscle cramps. They usually disappear after a few weeks.

• The medications can slow some people's heart rate, so an ECG is needed before starting the medication.

• A psychiatrist will review her regularly to monitor her progress on the medications, and this will include assessment of her memory using the mini-mental state examination.

What kind of support can we get?

• Community nurses can visit you and your wife on a regular basis to monitor the situation at home and will be able to advise you if the need arises.

• If your wife needs help with personal care, a home carer can visit and assist her. A social worker will work with you to make sure that both of you get the necessary help, including an occupational therapy assessment of the home (which may lead to home adaptations such as a stair lift) and the possibility of respite care.

• She can also be referred to a day hospital where her mental state can be monitored and she will be able to engage in group therapy.

• There are many organisations aimed at supporting patients and their carers in the UK, including the Alzheimer's Society and the Dementia Relief Trust.

15

Communication: Attention-deficit/ hyperkinetic disorder

Scenario: *A mother of a 7-year-old male recently diagnosed with attention-deficit hyperkinetic disorder (ADHD) wants to know more about the diagnosis. Address some of her concerns about her son's illness.*

Checklist of core knowledge

What is hyperkinetic disorder?
- Persistent pattern of inattention, hyperactivity, and impulsivity that is developmentally inappropriate.
  - Hyperactivity includes fidgeting, getting up and running about, excessive motor activity, and inability to play quietly.
  - Inattention includes decreased attention and getting easily distracted.
  - Impulsivity includes blurting out answers in class, inability to wait in line/take turns.
- Such behaviour must be present in two settings (e.g. home, school) for 6 months.
- Onset needs to be before the age of 7 years.
- Three times more common in male. Twice the risk in siblings.

What are the causes?
- Multifactorial, but some of the suggested causes include:
  - *Biological*: Imbalance of brain chemicals (noradrenaline, dopamine); genetic.
  - *Psychosocial*: Stress; difficulties in the family; poor attachment.

What treatments?
- Non-pharmacological treatments include cognitive behavioural therapy, parent management training, individual/family therapies, educational interventions.

- First-line drugs are stimulants, but these are only offered as part of comprehensive treatment for ADHD and should be prescribed by a specialist child and adolescent psychiatrist.

Methylphenidate (Ritalin): Stimulant that is most commonly used for ADHD

- This is not a cure, and only modifies the behaviours.
- *Mode of action*: Indirect sympathomimetic that increases release of dopamine and noradrenaline. It has a paradoxical effect to treat the symptoms.
- *Pre-treatment investigations*: Height, weight, blood pressure, and LFTs to be monitored regularly before and after commencing treatment.
- *Benefits*: They control the 'difficult behaviours' by increasing concentration and attention, while decreasing impulsivity. It is not a cure for ADHD.
- *Side effects*: Decreased appetite, anxiety, insomnia, tics, hypertension. At high doses, seizures have been reported. Long-term use of high doses may lead to growth suppression, and so 'drug holidays' (periods without medication) are needed.
- *Monitoring*: Patient should be under regular review by a specialist so that response can be monitored. If no response despite optimal titration, medication needs to be stopped. If improvement occurs and the patient becomes stable, treatment can be stopped at intervals to assess need for continued medication.

Prognosis

- May persist into adulthood, with hyperactive behaviours remitting early but inattention persisting; 20–30% will continue to have the full ADHD symptoms, and up to 60% may have one or more of the core symptoms.

16

Communication: Autism (pervasive developmental disorder)

Scenario: *The mother of a 5-year-old male has been informed that her child suffers from autism and thus she would like to know more about the illness. Address any concerns she may have.*

Checklist of core knowledge

What is autism?

- It is a developmental disorder that presents with problems in social interaction, communication, and repetitive behaviours and interests.
- Problems in social interaction mean that the individual may show little interest in forming peer relationships and sharing interests with others.
- Problems in communication may include delayed development of speech, unusual use of speech, and inability to initiate and sustain conversation with others.
- Repetitive behaviours include preoccupation with routines and rituals with restricted and unusual interests.
- It affects 5–10 people in 1000, and tends to affect boys four times more than girls.

Are there any other problems associated with autism?

- About 70% of children will have some degree of learning disability.
- Seizures are also more common.
- Behavioural problems are common and may include hyperactivity, temper tantrums, self-injury, and aggression.

What causes it?
- In most cases, the cause is unknown. In a few cases, the cause may be due to a genetic disorder such as fragile X or tuberous sclerosis.
- There is a small increase in the risk of having an autistic child if another child is affected.

Are there any treatments?
- There is no cure for the disorder.
- We help families cope by providing support, education, and sometimes family therapy.
- It is important that the child receives a statement of educational needs from a child psychologist. He may be able to remain at his current school with additional support or may benefit from attending a special school more suitable for his needs.
- A speech and language therapist can help him develop his language and communication skills.
- Children who present with difficult behaviour such as tantrums or aggression may benefit from behaviour therapy.
- Medication does not have a central role in the management of individuals with autism. It may be used to manage epilepsy, hyperactivity, and sometimes aggressive behaviour.

What is the prognosis?
- Prognosis seems to depend on IQ and the development of language.
- Most individuals will have significant lifelong problems, however about 10% of people work and live independently.

17

Communication: Antidepressant therapy with selective serotonin reuptake inhibitors

Scenario: *A 28-year-old female with a first episode of depression is about to be commenced on a selective serotonin reuptake inhibitor (SSRI), and wants to know more about it. Address any concerns she may have.*

Checklist of core knowledge

Why do I need an antidepressant?

- Antidepressants aim to prevent your depression from getting worse, and help you to get back to your normal self sooner.
- Roughly 70% of patients commenced on antidepressants will show some improvement.

How does it work?

- There are many types of antidepressants available, but they all work by altering the balance of brain chemicals called neurotransmitters. SSRIs stand for selective serotonin reuptake inhibitors, and they work on a chemical called serotonin.
- There may be some improvements after 2 weeks of treatment, but it takes roughly 4–6 weeks for the medication to have a full effect on you.
- It is important that you take the medication everyday.

What are the side effects?

- SSRIs are relatively safe with few side effects. However, some of the commonly reported ones are diarrhoea, nausea, vomiting, and restlessness. Most of these side effects go away after a few days.

• Some people have also experienced sexual problems such as decreased sex drive and difficulty having an orgasm, but remember that depression in itself can contribute to these problems as well.

How long do I need to be on them for?

• We usually recommend that you remain on antidepressants for at least 6 months once your depression goes away. When stopping, you will need to gradually reduce the dose of the medication rather than stopping abruptly.
• Antidepressants are not addictive, and you will not get dependence, tolerance, or cravings.

Are there other treatments other than antidepressants?

• Psychological treatments are available for the treatment for antidepressants. Cognitive behavioral therapy (CBT) is one of them, which attempts to change how you feel by changing the way you think.

Anything else I need to know?

• *Pregnancy*: It will be better for you to become pregnant after your episode of depression is over. We try to avoid medications in your first 3 months of pregnancy, but one has to weigh the pros and cons of doing so.

18
Communication: Lithium therapy

Scenario: *A 23-year-old female was admitted to hospital for a manic episode and was given a diagnosis of bipolar affective disorder. She has settled on the ward, and as part of her treatment, lithium therapy was suggested to prevent future relapses. She knows nothing about lithium and would like more information. Address any concerns she may have.*

Checklist of core knowledge

What is lithium?
- Lithium is a medication that has been in use for a very long time, and it is a very effective treatment for bipolar affective disorder (considered as 'gold standard'). It is also used as a 'mood stabiliser' in depression.
- We do not know the exact mechanism of action, but it appears to affect the way brain cells signal each other. (*Note*: It is thought to modulate secondary messenger systems, and affect ion permeability of neurons.)

How and when do I need to take it?
- Lithium comes in tablets, and you will need to take them every-day as directed. It is usually taken once a day (at night).
- Missing doses frequently may lead to relapses of your manic symptoms.

What are the side effects?
- *Short term*: Metallic taste, dry mouth, polyuria, polydipsia, mild tremor, lethargy, nausea and vomiting, diarrhoea, hair loss, benign leucocytosis.
- *Long term*: Weight gain, impaired renal function, hypothyroidism.

That sounds horrible. Is it really safe?
• Most of the side effects are related to the level of lithium in your body, and that is the reason why we monitor you closely while you are on lithium.
• Before we commence lithium therapy, we will conduct a full physical examination and a tracing of your heart (ECG). We will also do a blood test to check your blood count and make sure your kidneys and thyroid are working properly.
• Once you are on lithium, you will have regular blood tests (roughly every 3 months) to check the level of lithium in your blood. We will also check your kidney and thyroid at the same time.
• A safe level of lithium is between 0.4 and 1.0 mmol/L, and keeping lithium in this range will minimise any risk of side effects.

Are there any precautions I need to know about lithium?
• Lithium can interact with other medications (such as ACE-inhibitors, NSAIDs, SSRIs, antihypertensives) so you need to inform your doctor that you are on lithium. These medications can increase the lithium level in your body. Dehydration can also cause this.
• If you start feeling anxious, develop sudden tremors, have bloody diarrhoea, or become very lethargic, make sure you contact your doctor or go to hospital at once and get your lithium level checked to rule out lithium toxicity.
• Because lithium can affect the development of the foetus (e.g. cardiac malformation), make sure you use adequate contraception while on lithium. If in the future you decide to become pregnant, we will need to have a meeting to discuss your pregnancy and lithium therapy.
  – Lithium in pregnancy needs to be discussed to weigh the pros and cons of lithium therapy. Lithium is best avoided in the first trimester, as teratogenicity is highest.

19

Communication: Clozapine

Scenario: *A 36-year-old male with a diagnosis of schizophrenia is currently an inpatient in hospital. He was treated with risperidone and olanzapine but has not shown much improvement. The team decides to try clozapine treatment. Discuss this treatment with the patient with a view to obtaining consent.*

Checklist of core knowledge

What is clozapine?

- Clozapine is an atypical antipsychotic medication that has been shown to be very effective in treating psychotic symptoms in people with schizophrenia. Many people who previously did not respond to other antipsychotics seem to show good response to clozapine.
- It was first developed in the 1960s.

If it is so good, why wasn't I prescribed before?

- Unfortunately, clozapine does have side effects and so its use is currently limited to those who have been tried on two antipsychotics before (treatment-resistant schizophrenia). This is advocated by the UK NICE guidelines.

What are the side effects?

- The most serious side effect of clozapine is agranulocytosis, resulting in low white cell count (leucopenia, eosinophilia). This happens in roughly one out of 4000 patients. Platelet count can also decrease.
- It can also interfere with the heart, leading to arrythmias, myocarditis, and cardiomyopathy.
- Other side effects common to other atypical antipsychotics are also seen: anticholinergic (dry mouth, blurred vision), anti-adrenergic (hypotension), hypersalivation, weight gain.

Those side effects sound terrible.
Am I going to be alright on it?

• In order to ensure safety, we will carry out a full set of investigation before you start clozapine. This will involve a set of blood tests, including full blood count, and an ECG.

• All patients commenced on clozapine are then registered with the Clozaril Patient Monitoring Service (CPMS) to ensure that clozapine is given to you only if your blood result is at a safe level ('green' = OK, 'amber' = caution, 'red' = stop).

• We will start you on clozapine at the lowest dose (from 12.5 mg) and build up slowly to ensure that you are tolerating the medication. We will measure your vital observations regularly for the first few days. The usual dose we aim for is 200–400 mg a day.

You mentioned about regular blood tests
but how often is it?

• We will need to do your blood test every week for the first 18 weeks, but after this, it becomes every 2 weeks until 1 year. After that, it is monthly.

Anything I need to know while taking the
medication at home?

• You should not miss any doses. If you miss one dose, you can continue taking your regular dose from the next time. However, if you forget to take it for more than 2 days, you need to contact your doctor immediately as your dose will need to be re-titrated from the beginning again.

• If you experience any sore throat or fever while taking clozapine, you need to contact your doctor immediately.

20

Communication: Cognitive behavioural therapy

Scenario: *A 30-year-old female with depression is interested in psychological treatments for depression. She has heard of cognitive behavioural therapy (CBT) and approaches you for further information. Discuss the principles of CBT and the basic structure of therapy.*

Checklist of core knowledge

What is CBT?

- CBT helps individuals identify the links between thoughts, behaviours, and emotions. Our thoughts can influence how we feel and behave, and therefore we can change the way we feel by changing the way we think.
- It is a short-term treatment that usually lasts for 8–16 sessions and focuses on current problems rather than the past. Each session lasts for 50 minutes.
- CBT is usually performed by a psychologist but can also be performed by a psychiatric nurse, social worker, or psychiatrist.
- It focuses on the practical aspects of the given problem.

How does it work in depression?

- CBT is based on the idea that traumatic experiences in our childhood lead to the development of core beliefs that can be dysfunctional in some people. These core beliefs are the individual's 'rules for living' and determine how one behaves in certain situations. A stressful event can trigger off 'negative automatic thoughts', which are automatic thoughts that come into the person's head (e.g. 'it's my fault the company had gone bust') and these in turn can maintain low mood by making us less sociable, anxious, etc.
- The therapist helps the patient to identify and challenge these negative automatic thoughts, to break the vicious cycle, and helps the patient develop alternative ways of thinking.

What does it involve?

• An initial assessment is conducted to identify specific problems and goals.

• The therapist takes on an active role in the treatment, but the patient needs to be committed and motivated. This includes completing homework tasks.

• The patient is asked to keep a diary of situations that cause anxiety or depression and is asked to document the thoughts that he or she had at the time (thought record). By doing this the patient will be able to identify any negative automatic thoughts.

• The therapist helps the patient to challenge these negative automatic thoughts by looking at the evidence for and against these thoughts. 'Behavioural experiments' may be conducted to test out any misconceptions. Sometimes the patient is asked to schedule activities throughout the day and to rate these activities for pleasure (activity scheduling), which can help to improve mood.

• The end of the therapy will focus on strategies to prevent the individual from relapsing (relapse prevention work). Follow-up sessions are also offered.

What are the benefits of CBT?

• It can improve symptoms, identify factors that make one vulnerable to depression, and empower the individual to acquire techniques they can use in future problems.

• It has been shown to be as effective as antidepressants in mild to moderate depression, and results in a lower relapse rate than antidepressants. A combination of antidepressant treatment and CBT produces better results than either alone.

21

Communication: Electroconvulsive therapy

Scenario: *A 39-year-old male with treatment-resistant depression is admitted to hospital, and electroconvulsive therapy (ECT) was suggested as part of his treatment plan. Explain what the treatment involves and address any concerns the patient may have, with a view to consenting him for ECT.*

Checklist of core knowledge

What is it? Isn't it 'shock therapy'?

• ECT stands for electroconvulsive therapy, which is a treatment involving 'medically controlled seizures' using small electric currents. ECT has had a bad image in the past, but advances in treatment have made it a very safe treatment option.

What do you mean by medically controlled seizures?

• Before ECT, you will be given an anaesthetic to put you to sleep so you will not feel any pain during the treatment. You will also be given a medication to relax your muscles. An anaesthetist will be present during the treatment to monitor you.

• The psychiatrist will then put an electrode on your head (in the temples) and pass a small electric current, which will start the seizure. The seizures are thought to correct chemical imbalances in your brain, and this leads to improvement in your depression.

• After the treatment, you will be taken to a recovery room where a dedicated nurse will monitor your observations (blood pressure, pulse) and progress.

How often do I need this treatment?

• ECT is given roughly twice a week, and each course lasts between 8 and 12 treatments.

What are the benefits of ECT?
• It is an effective way of treating severe and treatment-resistant depression, and more than two-thirds of patients show improvement, usually within 2 weeks.
• It is often combined with antidepressants and other therapies.

What are the side effects? Can I die?
• Side effects from the complications of anaesthetic drugs can cause nausea, vomiting, muscle aches, and headaches on the day. ECT may also cause short-term memory problems, but these usually resolve completely.
• The risk of dying is very small (1 in 100,000), which is equivalent to someone dying from a general anaesthetic for a small operation (like getting a tooth taken out).

I'm not sure about ECT. Do I have to make up my mind now?
• We are not trying to pressure you into this treatment, and you do not have to make up your mind now. We want you to be fully informed before you make your mind up, so I want you to think about it and discuss with your friends and family.
• I can provide you with leaflets which will go over what we have discussed today, and we can set up another meeting to go through any questions you may have.

What happens if I refuse?
• If having fully understood all the information and you still feel strongly about not having ECT, we will respect your decision and we can explore other forms of treatment.
  – Note that this applies to patients who have the capacity to consent. For this, the patient must be able to fully understand the nature, purpose, and effect of the treatment, and the consequences of refusing it.

22
Communication: Detention under the Mental Health Act (1983)

Scenario: *A 23-year-old male was admitted to hospital under Section 2 of the 1983 Mental Health Act of England and Wales (MHA) because of a possible psychotic illness. Explain to him what compulsory admission under this act means.*

Checklist of core knowledge

Reasons for detention under the Mental Health Act
- *Criteria for the use of the act*: The person must be suffering from a mental illness of a nature and degree warranting admission to hospital, and there must be a risk to the health and safety of the patient or others.
- Compulsory detention is necessary to ensure the safety, protection, and treatment of patients with mental illness when they appear to lack the ability to look after themselves.

What is Section 2?
- Compulsory admission to hospital for the purpose of assessment. It is valid for 28 days.
- If a patient with a confirmed mental illness needs to be admitted against their will, Section 3 can be used. This is for treatment purposes and valid for 6 months.

Who is involved in putting a patient on a section?
- For both Sections 2 and 3, application by one approved social worker (ASW) and recommendations by two doctors are needed. One of the doctors must have specialist knowledge in treating

people with mental illnesses ('Section 12 approved'). Preferably one of the doctors will also have some knowledge of the patient.

Can the patient appeal against this?

- Patients can appeal to the hospital managers (through Hospital Managers Hearing), and/or to the Mental Health Review Tribunal. The tribunal is an independent panel consisting of a consultant psychiatrist, legal representative, and a lay member.

How can the patient be taken off a section?

- The patient's consultant (responsible medical officer), nearest relative, Hospital Managers, or the Mental Health Review Tribunal can.

Can a patient leave the hospital while on a section?

- No, but if their mental state improves, they can go off the ward temporarily as agreed with the consultant on Section 17 leave.

Any other information?

- Patients cannot be put on a section merely for carrying out treatments for physical illnesses that are not related to a mental illness.
- The Mental Health Act Commission ensures good practice of the Mental Health Act in hospitals.

23

Practical: Interpretation of blood tests

Scenario: *A patient treated in the community was recently commenced on lithium, and the results of her blood tests are: Serum lithium 1.9 mmol/L.*

Answer the following questions

1. What is the normal range for serum lithium levels?
2. Name two indications for using lithium in treating mental illnesses.
3. Name three investigations that need to be carried out prior to commencing a patient on lithium therapy.
4. How often should blood tests be carried out once serum lithium levels are stable?
5. How soon after taking lithium should bloods for serum levels be taken?
6. Name two medications that can interact with lithium.
7. Name two complications commonly seen with the serum lithium level given above.
8. Name two pieces of advice you would give to a patient with the serum lithium level given above.

Checklist of core knowledge

Normal range of serum lithium level
- The normal range differs between hospitals, but 0.4–1.0 is usually the standard range.

Indications of lithium therapy
- Treatment and prophylaxis of mania/hypomania, bipolar affective disorder, and recurrent depression.
- Augmentation therapy in treating depression.
- Aggressive or self-mutilating behaviours.

Pre-lithium investigations
• ECG.
• Thyroid function test.
• Renal function test (including urea and electrolytes).

Serum lithium monitoring
• Serum lithium levels are usually checked every 5–7 days until the levels are stable within the normal range. Once stable, they need to be checked every 3 months. (Renal and thyroid functions need to be checked every 6 months.)
• Blood tests for lithium levels are usually taken 12 hours after the last dose.

Some medications that can interact with lithium
• *Diuretics*: They can increase serum lithium levels by reducing its clearance. Thiazide interferes the most, while loop diuretics are relatively safer.
• *ACE-inhibitors*: They decrease the excretion of lithium.
• *NSAIDs*: These can increase serum lithium concentration by up to 40%.
• *Calcium channel blockers*: These can also increase serum lithium concentration.
• Increased neurotoxicity has been reported with *haloperidol, carbamazepine, and SSRIs*.

Lithium toxicity: occurs at levels greater than 1.5 mmol/L
• Early toxic effects are mainly gastrointestinal (anorexia, nausea, and diarrhoea) and CNS-related (restlessness, muscle weakness and twitching, tremors, ataxia, dysarthria, drowsiness).
• Above 2 mmol/L, marked disorientation, cardiac arrhythmias, and seizures are seen, with eventual progression to coma and death.

Advice to patient
• Stop taking lithium.
• Encourage adequate fluid intake.
• Seek urgent medical attention. In hospitals, steps are taken to reduce the serum lithium levels through intravenous rehydration, although haemodialysis can be used in cases of severe, life-threatening toxicity.

Further reading

The following is a list of core and advanced books that may be useful in supplementing your revision.

American Psychiatric Association. (2000) *Diagnostic and Statistical Manual of Mental Disorders DSM-IV*, Fourth Edition. American Psychiatric Association, Washington, DC.

Gelder M, Mayou R, & Geddes J. (2005) *Psychiatry*, Third Edition. Oxford University Press, Oxford.

Goldberg D & Murray R. (2006) *The Maudsley Handbook of Practical Psychiatry*, Fifth Edition. Oxford University Press, Oxford.

Katona C & Robertson M. (2005) *Psychiatry at a Glance*, Third Edition. Blackwell Publishing Ltd, Oxford.

Semple D, Smyth R, Burns J, Darjee R, & McIntosh A. (2005) *Oxford Handbook of Psychiatry*, First Edition. Oxford University Press, Oxford.

Sims A. (2003) *Symptoms in the Mind*, Third Edition. Saunders Publishing, Edinburgh.

Taylor D, Paton C, & Kerwin R. (2005) *The Maudsley 2005–2006 Prescribing Guidelines*, Eighth Edition. Taylor & Francis, London.

World Health Organisation. (1992) *The ICD-10 Classification of Mental and Behavioural Disorders: Clinical Descriptions and Diagnostic Guidelines*. World Health Organisation, Geneva.

Wright P, Stern J, & Phelan M. (2004) *Core Psychiatry*, Second Edition. WB Saunders, London.

Useful websites

The Mental Health Act Commission (http://www.mhac.org.uk)
The Misuse of Drugs Act (http://www.drugs.gov.uk)
National Institute for Health and Clinical Excellence (http://www.nice.org.uk)
The Royal College of Psychiatrists (http://www.rcpsych.ac.uk)
World Health Organisation (http://www.who.int/en)

Lightning Source UK Ltd.
Milton Keynes UK
UKOW03f1226300614

234282UK00001B/16/P

9 781405 175272